D1029067

what to eat
for how you feel

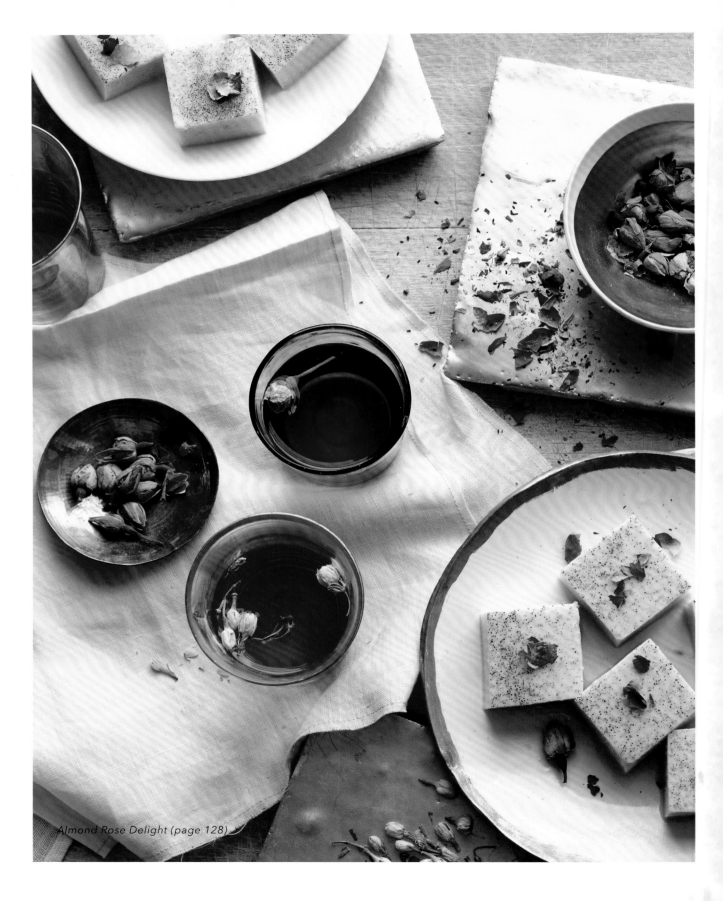

Almond Rose Delight (page 128)

THE NEW AYURVEDIC KITCHEN

what to eat
for how you feel

———

100 seasonal recipes

DIVYA ALTER

PHOTOGRAPHY BY
WILLIAM AND SUSAN BRINSON

RIZZOLI
NEW YORK

New York · Paris · London · Milan

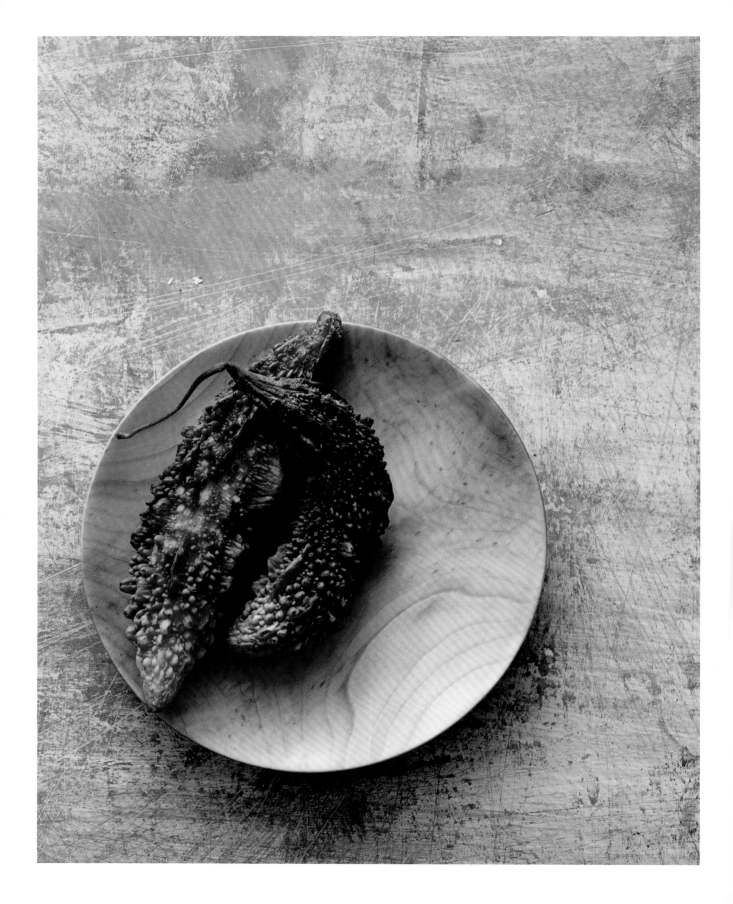

CONTENTS

OPPOSITE: *Bitter Melon*

FOREWORD

I'd never gone looking for Ayurveda, but somehow it found me and keeps finding me. And I'm so grateful for that.

As the authors of many best-selling books on gastronomy, my husband, Andrew Dornenburg, and I are often invited to speak at various venues across the country and around the world. Time and again, our visits would happen to coincide with a presentation on Ayurveda, this fascinating ancient system of natural healing that originated in India and that subsequently inspired both Tibetan medicine and traditional Chinese medicine.

Ayurveda's focus on health as the balanced integration of body, mind, and spirit intuitively struck me as wise. One of Ayurveda's key principles includes eating a flavorful diet, with every meal featuring it's six traditional tastes: sweet, sour, salty, bitter, pungent, and astringent. This system matches my own long-held belief of the importance of fully experiencing the flavor of our food—which can be seen metaphorically as the flavor of our lives—and to be truly conscious of it.

The insights I picked up along the way were enough to inspire me to share some of what I'd learned in my book *The Flavor Bible*, where I've included lists of "cooling" and "warming" ingredients that are useful to incorporate into dishes and drinks in the opposite weather conditions as a means of restoring balance to our bodies. So when our mutual friend chef Heather Carlucci, who owned New York City's acclaimed Northern Indian restaurant Lassi, introduced me via email to Ayurvedic expert Divya Alter, my curiosity was roused. Divya told me that she had found our books to be helpful to her in her work, and I was happy to learn that she'd even used and recommended them in the classes in Ayurvedic Nutrition and culinary training that she leads at Bhagavat Life, the school she and her husband, Prentiss, run in Manhattan.

Divya inspired me to learn more about Ayurveda, and I welcomed her offer to share the galleys for her first cookbook with me. Knowing what was coming didn't quite prepare me for what Divya has created in *What to Eat for How You Feel*. Divya's warmth and passion for her subject matter leap off every page and right into the reader's heart.

What to Eat for How You Feel provides a welcome overview of Ayurvedic principles for the uninitiated, and the timing of this book is perfect. Many are in desperate need of the lessons that Ayurveda has to offer, and after thousands of years in existence, Ayurveda seems to be reaching a tipping point where more and more people are opening to its worldview. America is in the midst of a health crisis—with the number-one cause of death being nutritionally controllable diseases. More than one out of three Americans is obese, and obesity contributes to several of the leading causes of preventable death, including heart disease, stroke, type 2 diabetes, and certain cancers. But regardless of weight, too many people don't know how to eat so their bodies can function properly and are able to heal from within. There are few more important lessons people can learn than to listen to their bodies and to provide them with the essential nourishment they need to keep them healthy and happy. This book provides important insights into a "modernized ancient" way of doing so.

The statistics bear out the fact that, at its worst, the wrong foods in the wrong quantities can be toxic to our bodies. But at its best, food is not only full of flavor; it also holds the power to transform us, uplift us, and heal us. Leading chefs around the globe are arriving at this realization. In 2014, renowned French chef Joël Robuchon declared that "The cuisine of the next ten years will be vegetarian." Subsequently, chef René Redzepi's Copenhagen restaurant Noma—widely considered one of the world's best restaurants—announced its plans to become a fully vegetarian restaurant during the spring and summer months. Many are finally coming to believe that the cuisine of the future will be a compassionate cuisine that is as healthful for our bodies and for the planet as it is delicious.

Divya—a Bulgarian yogini with equal passion for flavorful food and holistic healing—shares her firsthand knowledge of how Ayurvedic principles have helped her in her struggles with her own health challenges over the years. In doing so, Divya Alter chronicles food's powerful ability to transform our bodies and our health: physically, emotionally, mentally, and spiritually. She writes with the clarity of someone who has studied carefully and whose mastery of her subject spans the theoretical as well as the practical. Yet her words are always from the heart. As Divya tells her students, "Your love is the most important ingredient in everything you make."

Namaste, dear Divya, for offering your inspirational book as a gift to those looking to tap the healing power of food—deliciously. I'm so glad it found me.

—Karen Page, two-time James Beard Award–winning author of *The Flavor Bible* and *The Vegetarian Flavor Bible*

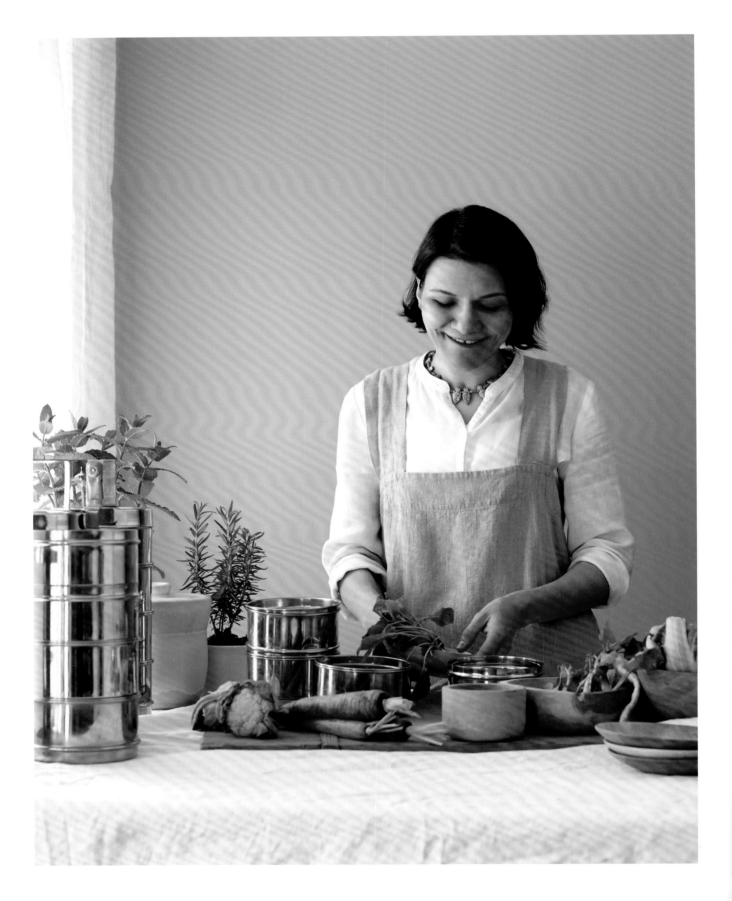

INTRODUCTION

For me, food is much more than a means of sustenance. It is a friend that has transformed and uplifted me on levels way beyond the physical.

My conscious relationship with food began when I started interning at the kitchen of an underground bhakti yoga ashram in my hometown of Plovdiv, Bulgaria. I grew up there during Communist times, when the government carefully monitored anything spiritual or religious. An awakening and rebellion in my late teens made me question life's purpose—Who am I? What is life all about? I searched for answers. Attracted to the yoga philosophy of India, I decided to become a yogini.

The problem was that in 1990 in Bulgaria, there were just a few books on yoga and no public yoga studios. I tried getting up before sunrise, taking a cold shower, and doing postures by looking at pictures—that lasted three days. I read that yogis choose a plant-based diet as a way to align with the practice of compassion and nonviolence. It made a lot of sense to me, but my mom and dad were in shock when I announced my decision to go vegetarian: "From tomorrow on, no meat, fish, and eggs!" "Then what's left to eat? Salads?" My parents had every right to be concerned, because I had no idea how to cook or how to be a healthy vegetarian.

Stubborn and determined, I kept searching until a friend took me to that underground ashram. It was a humble apartment with floor mats and cushions; a tiny altar was the only piece of furniture, yet I felt like I had stepped into a different world. The sparkling cleanliness, the charged yet calming energy, and the aromatic blend of incense and cooked food captivated my mind and senses. I was brought up as an atheist, but I kept thinking,

"There is something very spiritual about this place." After the yoga class, the three lovely hostesses served a feast of Indian vegetarian dishes that were so colorful, flavorful, and unbelievably delicious that I made my decision right then and there: "This is it. This is what I've been looking for."

At the time, I was just finishing high school; my parents wanted me to continue my education, but the college programs all seemed so boring to me. Instead, I decided to intern at the ashram. My first service was to wash pots and chop vegetables in the kitchen—this is how my journey of cooking and health began. My longing to connect with the roots of yoga took me to India, where I lived, worked, and studied for five years, and then to the United States, where I continued to study and eventually teach. Both in India and in the United States, personal healing crises led me to new discoveries and new teachers. Somehow Ayurveda, the traditional medicine of India, came into my life every time I searched for answers to how to improve my health and diet. My passion for Ayurvedic cooking turned into my occupation. Now, twenty-six years later, as a teacher myself, I am writing this cookbook!

Our relationship with food is infinitely personal, and it involves a lifetime of learning and practice. There's always something new to discover, something about it to understand better and spark fresh interest, ideas, and delight. Most of us start off our connection with food as something we eat and enjoy to satisfy hunger. However, there is so much more to learn from the food we eat. With *What to Eat for How You Feel*, I invite you to discover a new interaction with food by connecting with the healing properties of your ingredients, preparing them in ways that keep your digestion strong, and enjoying eating them, but also noticing how the food you eat makes you feel—immediately and in the long run. This is how food becomes your wisdom. I'd like to share a few lessons from my journey with the hope that you'll find some of them relevant to you.

THE KITCHEN IS A SACRED SPACE

My ashram mentors taught me to regard the kitchen as sacred. At first it was an intimidating place with the highest standards of cleanliness, punctuality, and restrictions on unrelated talking that I thought were extreme. In time, however, the kitchen became my favorite place, where I would welcome everything that uplifted me to a positive state of consciousness—whether it was the people, ingredients, music, or equipment. Food became my meditation.

While I was in India, I also learned how food can be a joyous part of life. India still has a pervading culture of food and hospitality, where dedicated mothers, sisters, wives, or daughters prepare fresh meals for family and guests, even in the hottest days of summer. I watched how the local people cooked each meal and sat down to eat together every day, and I saw firsthand how home-cooked meals become the nutritive foundation for supporting strong families, establishing lasting positive memories for children, and continuing family traditions. The friends and neighbors I learned local dishes from never gave me recipes; they just put a little bit of this and that into the pot and it always came out great. I learned that the best dishes are manifest in the hands of kind-hearted cooks who enjoy their passion and creativity in the kitchen, often without following a recipe. To date, food has helped me start long-lasting friendships.

HEALTH COMES FIRST

I learned from the teachings of A. C. Bhaktivedanta Swami, a prominent teacher in the bhakti yoga tradition, that a human being is born with three responsibilities:

1) **Maintain good health to stay alive.**

2) **Practice spirituality for personal growth.**

3) **Serve others, whether it is at home or at work.**

The body is our instrument with which we can offer our contributions to the world and attain spiritual perfection. I learned this lesson the hard way. For years I focused on my spiritual practice and serving others, while neglecting my personal needs. I put others first, and what, when, and how I ate came second. Gradually, my digestion weakened, and eating became my least favorite activity. My debilitated health turned into the biggest obstacle in my spiritual practice and my work—I could hardly do anything. It was during those painful moments of despair when I learned that health comes first, and healing begins with self-acceptance, self-compassion, and self-love; food is meant to keep us healthy, not to make us sick. For a while food was giving me so much discomfort that I thought food had turned into my enemy, but later food became a catalyst, leading me on a path of healing and discovery.

My studies in the United States included attending the Barbara Brennan School of Healing—yet another powerful period of personal transformation. Along with a comprehensive training in energy healing and psychology, I also learned about the importance of creating a healing team. Nowadays our health issues are so complex, with layers of underlying causes. We cannot expect one person, be it the most talented doctor, to address all our health needs. Over the years, I've had on my team healers, therapists, dentists, and physicians who helped me on different levels. And food became my research project. I started looking into the findings of modern nutrition and ancient medicine and learning how food could be used as medicine. I delved into Ayurveda, the traditional healing science of India, which I had been immersed in while living there.

SHAKA VANSIYA AYURVEDA– A Living Tradition of Healing and Cooking

In 2009, my husband, Prentiss Alter, and I moved to New York City, and I started teaching vegetarian cooking classes at Bhagavat Life, the educational nonprofit organization we had founded in 2006.

Despite my knowledge and practice of healthy eating and aggressive detoxification, my health worsened. I developed an auto-immune disorder, allergies, and chronic fatigue syndrome that lead to depression. Since modern medicine does not yet have a permanent cure for these illnesses, I searched for alternative treatments. Things finally shifted when I met Dr. Marianne Teitelbaum, an accomplished practitioner of Shaka Vansiya (SV) Ayurveda. I was very impressed by her approach, which differed from that of the contemporary Ayurveda I was familiar with.

Unlike contemporary Ayurveda, which is built on the limited ancient texts that survived the Mogul destruction, the knowledge and practice of SV Ayurveda was handed down through a familial lineage tracing back to ancient Vedic texts known as the Puranas. Today's application of SV Ayurveda healing protocols factors in our exposure to the many stressors of modern civilization that did not exist when the ancient texts were written such as electromagnetic frequencies, environmental pollution, depleted soil, toxic and processed food, and imbalanced

personal routines. One of the important ways it differs from contemporary Ayurveda is that many SV Ayurveda remedies are delivered and absorbed through the skin, bypassing the digestive system. With digestive conditions running rampant, this ensures that the remedies are absorbed properly and deliver the most effective treatment. In addition, SV Ayurveda doctors, who are also MDs, take the potential interaction of herbs and prescription medications into consideration in their treatment. This avoids any potential negative reactions and protects the patient from a healing crisis.

Dr. Teitelbaum's protocol included an SV Ayurvedic diet as a big part of my treatment, and gradually my inflammation and pain subsided and my energy levels started going up. As I was being treated, Dr. Teitelbaum introduced me to her teacher Vaidya R. K. Mishra, who is the successor in the ancient lineage of SV Ayurveda. With their treatment and the support from my healing team, today my autoimmune disease and allergies are completely gone. Food became my savior, and this is when I truly fell in love with food.

Vaidya R. K. Mishra was born in a family lineage of Ayurvedic doctors in India who preserved their medical knowledge even through the Mogul era, when most Ayurvedic Sanskrit texts were destroyed. Vaidya impressed me with his vast expertise in connecting the ancient texts with modern science. His ability to convey the secrets of his lineage beyond the boundaries of his family makes Ayurveda very practical and effective for us Westerners. Vaidya Mishra was the first to teach me not only the ancient theory of food, but also the hands-on skills of cooking it properly into delicious, light, and energizing meals. My years of training as a certified SV Ayurvedic practitioner culminated in developing systematic programs for Ayurvedic culinary education.

TURNING COOKING
INTO A CAREER

Among the many great chefs I interned with, I was fortunate to learn in person from Yamuna Devi, the award-winning author of *Lord Krishna's Cuisine: The Art of Indian Vegetarian Cooking* and *Yamuna's Table*. She was such a remarkable person! The first lesson Yamuna Devi taught me was the first lesson she learned: before you begin cooking, remember your teachers with respect. We've all met teachers, whether in school or in life, who helped us be better and do better. Why not remember them in the kitchen? Yamuna would do that by singing a Sanskrit mantra, and ever since, so do I. Food became one way for me to express love and gratitude.

Over the past eight years in New York City, cooking has turned into my career—teaching cooking classes, hosting dining events, providing catering and meal delivery service, managing the kitchen, launching the first in the world professional Ayurvedic chef's training program, starting a restaurant—only veteran chefs will understand what Prentiss and I got ourselves into! We love what we do, and we are thrilled when our students and clients come back to us telling us how the little things they've learned at our school contributed to small or big changes in their lives. Food became my way of reaching out to the world.

STARTING A CONSCIOUS
RELATIONSHIP WITH FOOD

A conscious relationship with food begins with getting to know each other. In the same way that the people we hang out with shape our mind-set and lifestyle, the foods we choose to put in our bodies shape our physical and mental strength. But then why does the same healthy food have different effects on different people? Why is it that when you and I eat the same salad, you feel boosted and I feel bloated? How do I figure out what foods are good for me? How do I prepare them with spices to enjoy nourishing, enlivening meals without unpleasant side effects?

If like me, you have searched and asked these questions, I hope you will find answers in *What to Eat for How You Feel*. I wrote this book to share the excitement and sense of possibility my students and I experience in our encounters with pure, sumptuous food at home. This is not the new diet book. I believe that one's personal diet has to correspond to one's unique needs, and needs change constantly. *What to Eat for How You Feel* is an attempt to teach you the principles by which you can link your physical and mental needs with the foods and seasonings that will balance you accordingly. When people ask me to describe Ayurvedic food, my answer is: whatever your definition of healthy food is fresh, pure, seasonal, local, predominantly plant based, nutrient rich, easy to digest, satisfying, energizing, healing, balancing selected and prepared according to your individual needs.

MY APPROACH TO COOKING
WITH AYURVEDA

Now a few words about my Ayurvedic approach to food, cooking, and the organization of this book. I have sifted through and synthesized a great deal of knowledge and recipes that I've learned largely during my years of study and practice of SV Ayurveda. This ancient wisdom has been preserved and practiced for thousands of years in India, but cooking with it does not have to be limited to Indian cooking. With my diverse recipes I offer you practical ways to bridge the gap between the ancient wisdom of food and modern living beyond the boundaries of India. Whether you prepare Asian-style Stir-Fried Red and Black Rice, Italian-style Spinach Risotto, or French-Style Braised Root Vegetables, you will still be cooking Ayurvedic food. Why? Because you will be applying the ancient principles of selecting high-quality ingredients and combining and preparing them in ways that are compatible for your type of digestion.

Instead of looking at foods as mixtures of different chemicals, Ayurveda looks at foods as combinations of the five physical elements—space, air, water, fire, earth—and how these food elements and their qualities interact with the same elements and qualities in our physiology. Digestion is the central mechanism that transforms food molecules into energy and our bodily tissues, and influences our thoughts and feelings. As our digestion fluctuates with changes in the weather, I've organized the recipes according to season and offer recipe variations according to one's strength of digestion. The recipes in *What to Eat for How You Feel* will free you from the distraction of having to guess or experiment or analyze as you prepare a personalized meal. At the same time, giving thought and analysis to my explanations will gradually free you from the necessity of following recipes and will help you deal with the unexpected.

If there are ingredients in my recipes you've never used, welcome the opportunity to try something new. The challenge of finding pure and nutritionally potent ingredients that address the widespread health issues of allergies, inflammation, and digestive and autoimmune disorders motivated me to become innovative. I've created familiar yet unexpectedly delicious dishes that bring new forms of pleasure to the table for a sustained healthy diet. My goal is to show you how to apply Ayurvedic principles to any cuisine. To my many chef colleagues who value the healing approach to their craft and look for ways to respond to the growing demand for appealing gluten-free and dairy-free vegetarian alternatives, check out my Almond Milk Béchamel Sauce (page 188), Lasagna with Broccolini, Carrots, and Spinach (page 112), and Raisin-Cranberry Sauce (page 117). Although all recipes are lacto-vegetarian, you don't have to be a vegetarian to cook with *What to Eat for How You Feel*. We all need to eat our vegetables!

For decades, I've welcomed thousands of people into my kitchen. From the novice, whose main culinary skill was to boil water without burning it, to the professional cook who wanted to know about the healing benefits of ingredients, I've learned that anyone can become a confident, health-conscious cook, and that fresh, seasonal food can make you feel better and do better for the world. I offer this book to my teachers and students who continuously inspire me to grow and give, and to anyone who, like me, has been searching for healthier ways to eat and to make friends with food.

The ancient Vedic texts of India state that our whole body is built around two things: the food that comes into the mouth and the words that come out of the mouth—both must be healthy and harmonious for the well-being of ourselves and others. I sincerely hope that the words coming out of my mouth (or mind) that strung together this book will inspire you to put the best food in your mouth. Healthy food promotes healthy thoughts, conversations, and relationships that ripple into sustaining healthy families, communities, and societies.

Om tat sat.

PART ONE

OUR RELATIONSHIP WITH FOOD

THE AYURVEDIC PERSPECTIVE

IS ALL HEALTHY FOOD HEALTHY FOR *YOU*?

A PERSONALIZED APPROACH TO EATING

Running Bhagavat Life, our Ayurvedic culinary school in New York City, I've met thousands of amazing people over the years. When I ask my students to talk about their relationship with food, most of them tell me that they are trying to eat healthier. What does that really mean, and how can Ayurveda help them do that?

Modern technology makes food knowledge more accessible than ever, but how usable is all that information? There's a barrage of often contradictory opinions about healthy foods, eating habits, and diets. You've probably experimented with a few of them yourself—some worked for you and some didn't. Have you tried a famed super food that didn't sit well with you? Or have you taken to a diet that made you feel better for a time but later turned against you? Does your roommate swear by Paleo or raw food, but does your stomach just say no?

As a chef and nutritionist myself, I've gone through tests and trials with food for many years, but somehow I never felt I was getting the full package. I finally felt satisfied when I learned about Ayurveda and grasped the explanations that tradition provides—they just made the most sense to me, and when I put them into practice, they worked. Ayurveda is the oldest and most comprehensive healing science known to humankind, dating back more than five thousand years.

I was introduced to it in India while I was being treated for a severe digestive disorder by an Ayurvedic doctor. The doctor told me that there is no good or bad food in itself. A food or herb can be good for someone or bad for someone—it depends on one's individual needs at that time. As I kept asking him, "What about this?" or "What about that?" his answer, every time, was "It depends!"

I was really impressed by how my treatment protocol included food as medicine and how none of the therapies or remedies I was given had any side effects. Being a trained vegetarian cook, I decided to study the food guidelines of this ancient science and tap into the subtle, healing aspects of food that modern nutrition is still discovering. Life took me to the United States, where I was fortunate to not only marry my husband, Prentiss, but also meet my primary Ayurvedic teacher, Vaidya R. K. Mishra, successor in the age-old tradition of Shaka Vansiya (SV) Ayurveda. Unlike any other doctor I've met, Vaidya Mishra is also an expert cook who was raised on Ayurvedic food. In *What to Eat for How You Feel* I'm excited to share with you the secrets and practical aspects of Ayurvedic cooking from his lineage that work for us today.

To this day, I am fascinated by how the oldest written knowledge in the world can still be relevant to us. How did the ancients know that turmeric is anti-inflammatory without testing it in a lab? How did they figure out there were friendly bacteria in the gut and that their deficiency caused problems all over the body? I look forward to modern science

proving true more of the universal principles of health described in the ancient medical texts. In the meantime, I want to share with you my experience of applying these universal principles to your food today. I hope *What to Eat for How You Feel* will help you understand the connection between the two and how to choose the foods that will balance you. Selecting the ingredients that are right for you and preparing them properly are the first steps to making cooking and eating healthy as well as enjoyable.

From the Ayurvedic texts to the Daoist classics of Chinese medicine to the writings of Hippocrates, all classical medical texts encourage us to regard food as medicine. How did doctors treat their patients up until 150 years ago, when pharmaceutical drugs did not yet exist? It was through herbs, foods, and regimens that assisted the body in healing itself. I doubt that even the most advanced medical drugs and practices will completely cure a patient without addressing the necessary changes in diet. You can have the best doctor prescribe the best medicine for you, but if you eat poor quality food, your healing can be very slow, if even possible. Eating the food that's right for you will create the favorable conditions for your body and mind to thrive, to be full of life.

"Without proper nutrition, medicine is of little use. . . . With proper nutrition, medicine is of little need."
—CHARAKA SAMHITA, an ancient classical text on Ayurveda

Food = Energy

Ayurveda defines life as the uninterrupted flow of *prana*, or the life-giving cosmic energy in the body; death is the cessation of that flow. The role of food is to charge us with energy, or prana, but why is it that sometimes we eat and feel awake and energized, and other times we feel totally drained and need to take a nap? Depending on how our digestion interacts with the quality, freshness, and method of preparation, foods give us different pranic charges—some foods are full of life, and others are energetically dead.

Before we move on, let us assess the food we eat daily from a different angle than we usually do—is it invigorating, lackluster, or depleting?

Foods that **invigorate** us, that bring us a bright charge of prana, are freshly prepared and seasonal, locally grown in nutrient-dense, toxin-free soil. When such foods are properly combined in recipes and prepared appropriately so that their vital nutrients are preserved, in a positive, loving environment, we digest them perfectly, feeling energized and balanced, nourished down to a cellular level. Our systems eliminate on time, our natural healing capacities are supported, and our life may be prolonged—and most of all, we feel happy.

Some foods are **lackluster**, not bright with energy. Think about leftovers or frozen foods—their fresh energy is long gone. Other lackluster foods are those that are hard to digest or combined to disadvantage in recipes. They don't shine! They may taste pleasant at first but cause us digestive discomfort later. And we feel lackluster after eating when we eat in a hurry, under stress, or when we eat food prepared without care in a negative environment. Eventually, a steady diet of this type of food can produce a variety of mild digestive disorders.

Depleting foods are drained of energy—and they can drain us too. Canned, deep-fried, microwaved, heavily processed, and artificial foods, and sometimes even slightly rotten or putrefied foods, may taste like food, but they give us no prana. They clog the body's digestive system, elimination systems, and even its subtle channels of energy, and a steady diet of such foods leads to imbalance and disease. Imagine that you're standing in front of a peach tree, its branches bending with sweet, juicy, aromatic fruit at your grasp, and I passed by and offered you a can of peaches—which will you pick, the fruit off the tree or the can?

I do not have to convince you that invigorating food is healthy food. It is what we need to eat to live optimally and maintain harmony with nature. Unfortunately, the modern lifestyle promotes the convenience of packaged and processed foods that are far from invigorating. Famous chefs and popular food bloggers teach us "intelligent" ways of eating leftovers, disregarding the high health cost of leftovers: they give us less energy and weaken our digestion, thus leading to illness. What can we do when eating invigorating food takes a lot of work and eating lackluster and depleting food is convenient and affordable?

If you found your meals fall more into the last two categories, do not despair! As you build your awareness of the quality of the food you put in your mouth, I hope you will gradually move from less depleting and lackluster food and to more invigorating meals. Eating invigorating food all the time is ideal, but it might not be realistic for your current situation. When your real situation is not the ideal, at least you can try the next best: occasionally eating lackluster food is better than eating depleting food. Even if you don't change anything in your diet, by simply making an effort to include more freshly prepared meals, your energy levels will surely go up. The more invigorating food you eat, the more your immune system will act intelligently and do its job of keeping you strong.

In my experience, well-being is a participatory process—if you want to feel well, you have to do well, or do better, not only with your diet but also with your lifestyle and your environment. Good diet, routine, and environment are the three pillars of health that support our integration on physical, mental, emotional, and spiritual levels. Whenever you feel off-track, go back to the basics of proper nutrition. What you eat is often easier to change than how and where you live. Sustaining a healthy diet will give you the strength and determination to make necessary adjustments to your routine and environment when the time is right.

Finding Your Alignment

We all want to be healthy, but health alone is hardly anyone's purpose of life. A healthy body is an instrument with which we can fulfill our dreams and offer our contributions to the world. In the words of one of my teachers, Jayadev Singh, "If you have a mind, you have a mission. What is your mission and how well is it activated?" We need to align what we eat, how we live, and where we are with what we are meant to do in this life. The more aligned we are, the more we experience a deep sense of fulfillment and long-lasting happiness.

One of my passions in life is to receive and share knowledge. The kitchen is my sacred space where I like to spend quiet moments of meditative cooking and recipe creation; it is my workspace of heat, noise, and heavy-pot lifting in service to others; and it is my classroom full of fun and joy as I witness people discover something new about their relationship with food. Sharing knowledge gets a bit more challenging with close family, but I've had success with teaching my egg-free muffin recipe to both my eighty-year-old father-in-law, Nick, who is a fantastic cook, and my six-year-old niece, Carla, who cannot read yet and had never baked before. I love to assist people in learning what I am good at—cooking healthful meals.

Steeped in thousands of years of wisdom, the principles and practice of cooking I present here, although based on SV Ayurveda, are universal and simple enough to follow, even for those who are too busy or too tired to cook. No matter what culture we live in, what our religion and beliefs are, what we do or who we hang out with, one aspiration unites us: we all could eat healthier. Nourishing ourselves with real, clean, vibrant foods will unlock our vitality and enhance our ability to transform from within. It has worked for countless of people through the ages, and it works for me. I believe it can work for you too.

ARE YOU MOSTLY AIRY, FIERY, OR EARTHY?

CONNECTING YOUR FOOD CHOICES WITH YOUR DIGESTION

As long as you are in a human body, you've got to deal with the building blocks of all creation, which the ancients defined as space, air, fire, water, and earth, the five physical elements that manifest in the body in different ways. For example, Ayurveda holds that our tissue layers and bones have a great amount of earth, the body fluids represent water, the metabolism is a manifestation of fire, and all movement in the body is carried out by air. In a poetic sense, the human body is earth, water, fire, and air moving through channels of space.

When discussing body-mind constitutions, Ayurveda lists the combinations (aka *doshas*) of these elements like this:

space + air = Vata

fire + a little water = Pitta

water + earth = Kapha

Every individual has these combinations in different proportions—that's one reason each person is unique—and the proportions can go up or down depending on the season or surrounding circumstances. Some people are more airy (Vata), some are more fiery (Pitta), and others more earthy (Kapha). This is why one food or herb cannot be good or bad for everyone—it may be good or balancing for one, but toxic and aggravating for another. Or an herb may be good for you in this season but may not work for you in another.

Figuring out your constitution takes a lot more than answering a "dosha quiz"—you need an expert Ayurvedic doctor to read your pulse. But knowing your constitution is not enough to stay healthy; you also need to know what your imbalance is. During my studies of contemporary Ayurveda, I often felt confused: if I have a Vata-Pitta body type but one day I feel very heavy and congested (Kapha imbalance)—what am I supposed to eat then? I was never sure how to resolve the complexity of eating according to my constitution while at the same time addressing seemingly opposing imbalances. I struggled with similar contradictions until I started studying the Shaka Vansiya Ayurveda tradition, which made it clear and very practical for me: eat seasonally, according to the strength of my digestion and how I feel overall today. This is why I decided to group the recipes in this book according to harvest season and give variations for each recipe based on the strength of your digestion, so that you can cook healthy food even if you have no knowledge of Ayurveda.

We live in a world of polarities—for every positive charge there is a negative, for every feminine aspect there is a masculine, for every up there is a down. According to the same principle, every element has energy, and every energy has its own particular attributes, or vitality-enhancing qualities, as well as challenges, which can cause weakness or disease. With Ayurveda, we can strengthen the attributes and diminish the challenges of each element.

The following charts outline some common manifestations of our Airy, Fiery, and Earthy qualities, color-coded in their transformation from attributes to mild imbalances to serious challenges. Before turning to the recipes and choosing meals, ask yourself: Do I feel more Airy, Fiery, or Earthy today? The recipes have information about working with each of the three aspects.

As you study the characteristics of each type, please do not focus on what's wrong with you (or others) when you identify with some of the challenges. You should expect some anxiety or some gas, some anger, or laziness once in a while—that's natural for all of us. Our mind-set should be to continuously balance these mild and transient challenges to prevent them from becoming consistent and chronic.

It is good to understand the challenges for educational purposes, but dwelling on them will drag your mind down. Elevate yourself by looking for the assets in you or another individual; relate to whatever is uplifting about you and others. Find the positive charge in the negative expression.

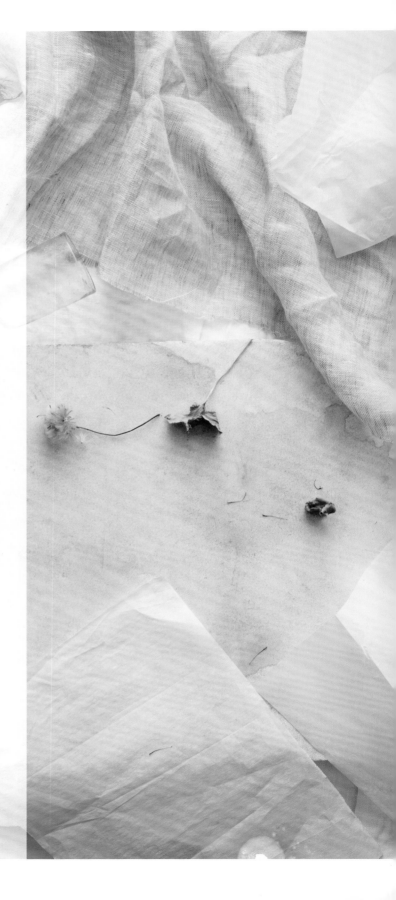

THE AIRY

Think about what air is like: cold, dry, and light, moving quickly all over the place.

Air supports all motion, catabolism (breaking down of molecules to release energy), and elimination; it helps you perceive touch and makes your mind fast and quick to grasp knowledge. Through your Airy nature you uplift others with your divine lightness and angelic presence.

When aggravated, the same energy of air can throw you off. Are you feeling overly active, nervous, cold? Do you experience Airy type digestive problems: bloating, gas, burping, constipation? Does your mind race, and do you feel like you don't have time to fully process your thoughts, desires, and feelings? Another mark of too much air is experiencing the "colder" emotions: fear, worry, anxiety. When your airs move too fast, you rush into everything you do; your life seems "up in the air."

Airy qualities are also accentuated in fall-winter and during the elder stage of life.

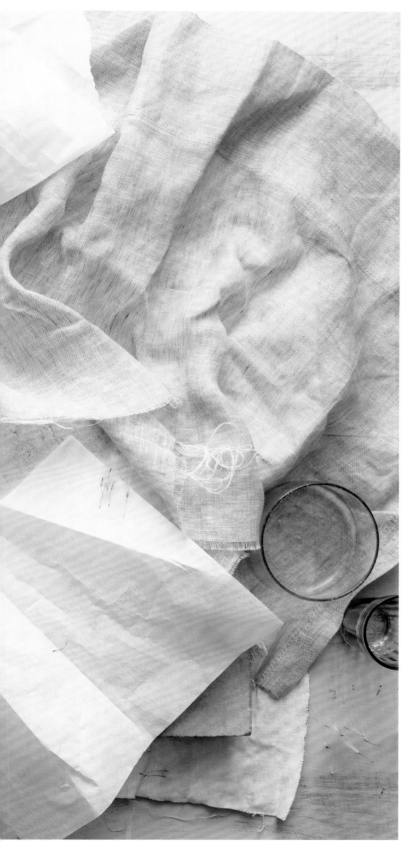

ATTRIBUTES	MILD IMBALANCES	CHALLENGES
Slender	Unwanted weight loss	Emaciated
Cooler body temperature	Cold hands and feet	Catches cold easily
Drier skin and hair	Scaly skin, dandruff	Wrinkles, dry eczema
Irregular meals	Irregular appetite	Loss of appetite
Sensitive stomach	Gas, hiccups, bloating	Chronic constipation
Light sleeper	Scary/active dreams	Insomnia
Active	Hyperactive	Worn down
Creative	Absentminded, scattered	Can't materialize ideas
Enthusiastic	Mood swings	Short-term depression
Bursts of energy	Low stamina, fatigue	Chronic fatigue
Loves change	Unsteady, frivolous	Unregulated
Sensitive/ intuitive	Bothered by noise and smell	Hypersensitive
Communicative	Talkative	Babbling
Easily excited	Restless	Anxious
Extroverted	Insecure, fearful	Panic attacks
Cheerful	Unstrung	Nervous breakdown

The Grounding recipes on
pages 143 to 183 and the variations
for Airy digestion in the recipes
throughout the book will help you a
great deal with calming the Airy
storms in your body (and life).
In general, when you feel "up in the air,"
your mantra is "Slow down and breathe!"
Keep repeating it to yourself
and find ways to connect with the
calming, nurturing, stable energy
of Mother Earth.

THE FIERY

Picture fire. It is hot, oily, unstable, stimulating, drying, penetrating, and when ablaze, it is difficult to temper. The fire energy impels action, produces heat, and brings about transformation. It gives you the sense of perception, illumination, purpose, passion, and radiance. Through our Fiery nature we uplift others with our divine brightness.

Just like turning up the heat changes sensation from comfortably warm to burning hot to destructive, when your fiery energy goes up, you begin to experience "burning" physical sensations: your radiant skin turns reddish and is affected with acne, eczema, or brown spots; your bright eyes turn reddish and dry. You experience "burning" digestive problems: unsatiated appetite, hyperacidity, heartburn. Your sharp, insightful, and focused mind becomes unstable, and if someone pushes your buttons, you erupt into the "hot" emotions of anger, jealousy, and impatience. You are on fire!

Fiery qualities are also accentuated in summer and from adolescence until advancing age.

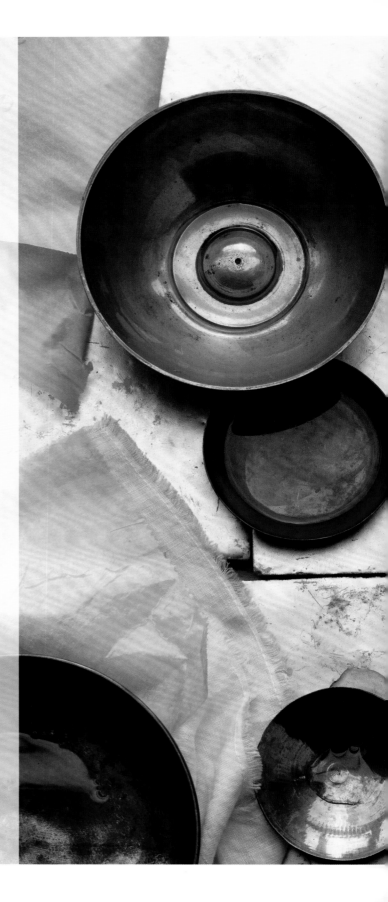

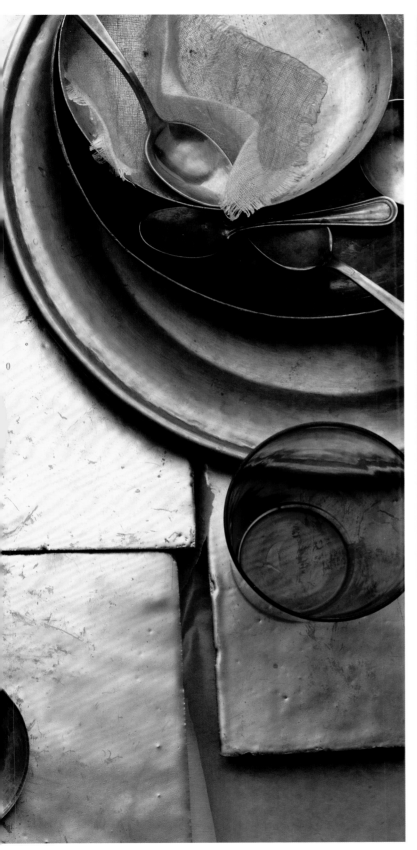

ATTRIBUTES	MILD IMBALANCES	CHALLENGES
Strong digestion	Excessive hunger and thirst	Acid reflux, ulcers
Radiant skin	Skin redness, rosacea	Acne, psoriasis
Warmer body temperature	Hot flashes, excessive sweat	Inflammation, fever
Righteous	Rigid	Dishonest, corrupt
Trusting	Cynical, doubtful	Does not trust anyone
Sharp intellect	Sarcastic, critical	Judgmental, manipulative
Persistent	Impatient	Excessive, addicted
Precise	Perfectionist	Nit-picker
Courageous	Takes unnecessary risks	Foolhardy
Passionate	Lustful	Overly stimulated
Ambitious	Pushy	Aggressive
Protective	Possessive	Jealous, controlling
Dynamic, energetic	Forceful, impulsive	Overdoing everything
Emotional	Temperamental, irritable	Angry, violent
Natural leader	Bossy	Goes on power

The Cooling Recipes on
pages 96 to 135 and the variations
for Fiery digestion in the recipes
throughout the book will offer you
immense relief in taming your fires.
In general, when you feel like a
firecracker, your mantra is "Chill out!" Keep
repeating it to yourself as you
find ways to connect with the cooling,
calming energy of water and earth.

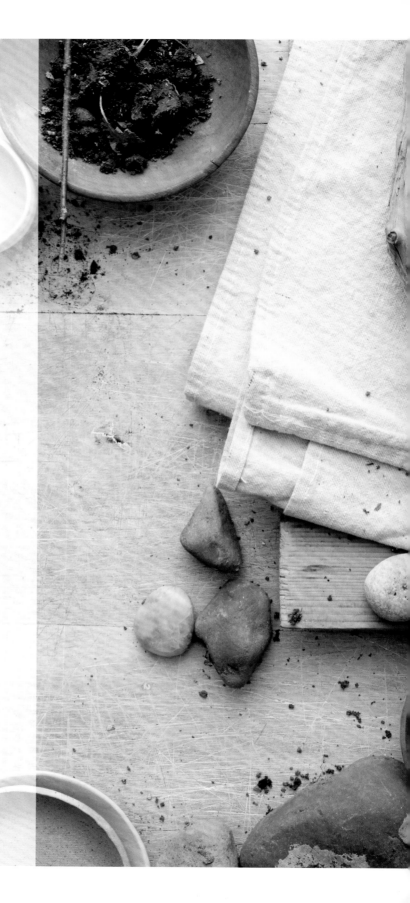

THE EARTHY

Visualize the earth. It's massive, solid, stable, heavy, cool. It is our source of nourishment and sustenance, and it contains vast water reservoirs that provide us with moisture and fluidity. The earth element in the body creates and supports its structure and growth (anabolism), and the water element (or fluids) lubricate and nourish every cell. Through your earthy nature you uplift others by your divine nurturing presence.

With the power of your earthiness you remain calm and patient, steady and enduring, loving, devotional, and accepting. You feel strong, secure, and stable. But when your earthiness overwhelms your balance, you build up excessive tissue and gain weight, become congested, take too long to make changes in your life. You experience sluggish digestion. You dwell in the "heavy" emotions: depression, sadness, lethargy. You feel stuck.

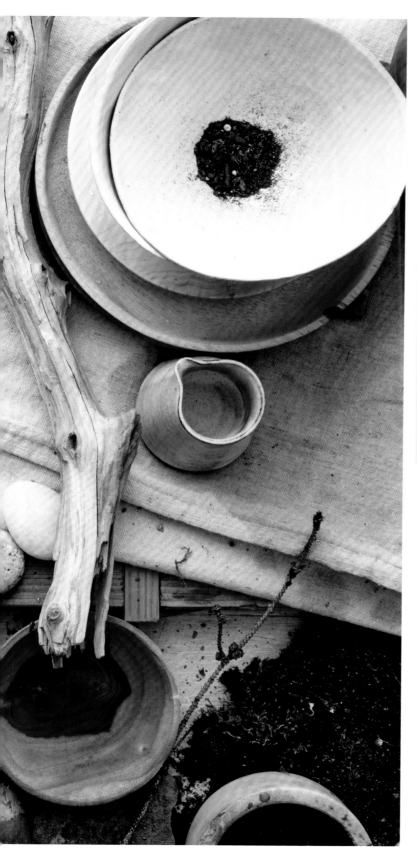

ATTRIBUTES	MILD IMBALANCES	CHALLENGES
Strong	Dense, stiff muscles	Physical weakness
Moist, supple skin	Oily, puffy skin	Wet eczema
Well-lubricated tissues	Swelling	Water retention, bloating
Thrives in warm, dry climate	Colds and flu	Congestion, asthma
Caring and compassionate	Compromising	Apathetic
Long-term memory	Begrudging	Can't let go
Slow but steady	Delays things	Procrastinates
Sound sleeper	Sleeps too much	Lazy
Content	Complacent	Egoistic
Loyal, devotional	Unable to say no	Fanatical
Loves routine	Fearful of change	Stagnation

The Energizing Recipes on pages 56 to 89 and the variations for slow digestion in the recipes throughout the book will give you a good kick to shake off your piled-up earthi-ness. In general, when you feel heavy like a mountain, your mantra is "Let go and move on!" Keep repeating it to yourself as you find ways to connect with the light, mobile energy of air and the transformational energy of fire.

WHAT TYPE OF DIGESTION DO YOU HAVE?

The mechanics of the initial stage of our digestion are very similar to cooking food in a pot. Imagine that your stomach is a pot cooking on the stove of your digestive system. Strategically placed in the center of our body, the stomach is one of the main transformers and distributors of the energy we receive through food. Just like a gas burner is connected to pipes supplying fuel and has gaps allowing a flame to go through, the stomach is connected to channels or "pipes" that carry the fuel (Pitta) produced from the food we ate yesterday. When we eat, the food goes into that stomach pot, the metabolic fire composed of various acids and enzymes turns up, and your meal starts cooking. The gastric juice is the liquid that prevents the food from burning, and the air in the stomach helps with peristalsis, moving the food around to break it down. The innate intelligence of the body regulates the strength of the flame in the same way that we constantly adjust a stove's heat depending on what we are cooking.

We all digest food differently. As we've discussed earlier, the strength of your digestive fire is one of the most important factors in determining what foods are healthy for you. Ayurveda describes four main types of digestion: balanced, irregular (Airy), sharp (Fiery), and slow (Earthy).

In a **balanced** state, your flame burns neither too high nor too low, and you enjoy a healthy appetite; after a meal, you feel satiated and blissful. Your optimal digestion, absorption, and elimination are attuned with the needs of your body. It's like cooking your food to perfection.

Unfortunately, stress, processed foods, leftovers, bad food combinations, and unhealthy eating habits can take our digestion off balance. **Irregular, Airy digestion** usually occurs when too much air in the stomach makes the digestive fire sometimes high, sometimes low, and appetite fluctuates. It's like cooking on a gas stove with a fan blowing into the flame and making it waver too much—your food will end up unevenly cooked. Irregular digestion often produces Airy-type reactions such as flatulence, bloating, constipation, dryness, and belching without acidity. The toxic residue from the semi-digested food can potentially make us experience fatigue, stiffness, and poor circulation.

Sharp, Fiery digestion occurs when the fire in the stomach is turned up too high. Imagine sautéing vegetables in a pan with barely any water on the highest heat without stirring. Gradually the food will dry and burn, making it inedible. Similarly too high "fire" can reduce moisture in your stomach, causing some nutrients and friendly bacteria to burn before they reach the state of absorption—you end up always feeling hungry, craving more food, especially sweets, but losing weight and experiencing nutrient deficiency. Eating a lot of Fiery foods when you have sharp Fiery digestion may result in burning reactions such as hyperacidity, heartburn, dryness, bad breath, gastritis, and ulcers. Fiery digestion often produces hot, acidic toxicity that can potentially trigger inflammation.

Slow, Earthy digestion is just the opposite of the Fiery—it occurs when the digestive flame is too low and there is more dampness in your stomach. It's like trying to boil food in a lot of water on the lowest heat—it takes forever. Slow digestion is often caused by eating food without spices or by blockages in some of the "gaps" of the stomach—the flame simply does not come through. As such, your stomach cannot fully break down the food you eat. With slow (Earthy) digestion you may experience the heavy type of digestive problems: sluggishness, fatigue after eating, loss of appetite, congestion, lack of circulation, weight gain.

Note: If you experience severe symptoms of any type of digestion, consult with a medical doctor without delay.

Seasons also affect our capacity to break down food completely. It is quite likely that many of us will experience irregular, Airy digestion during late fall and early winter, sharp, Fiery or irregular, Airy digestion during late winter and summer, and slow, Earthy digestion during spring. Understanding how the seasonal changes affect our bodies will help us make balancing food choices.

Optimal health is only possible when we enjoy balanced digestion consistently.

FINDING BALANCE IN YOUR DIET

Take a moment to comprehend the marvelous, divine ways in which the elements in nature move. Energy is never static—it flows, ripples, and swirls in rhythms and cycles that we may perceive as harmonic or chaotic—but the constant movement of energy gravitates toward one universal state: balance. Balance is never static either—it involves continuous adjustments. The invisible law behind it all is "Like increases like, and opposites balance."

The desire for balance is inherent to all; it is our foundation for peace and happiness. However, each one of us has a unique reference point for balance, based on the body-mind constitution we were born with—this is what we want to come back to when we're seeking optimal health. According to Ayurveda, by understanding our reference point for balance, we will know how to keep equilibrium between our physical and emotional tendencies in relation to the external world.

Part of our complex human existence is our balance "security system" that alarms us when things go off. It could be adjusting your sitting posture to get rid of a cramp, or

putting on a sweater when you feel cold, or taking it easy after a long day of work—these things we do automatically are all ways to find balance. If we neglect the alarm signals, an unchecked imbalance will make the five elements deviate from their natural proportions, and we feel unwell or even develop an illness. Unfortunately, once we are in a more imbalanced state, we tend to crave or select things that will perpetuate the imbalance rather than those that will soothe it. It's like feeling very Fiery but craving spicy, bold foods despite an inevitable burning discomfort after the meal. When you find yourself trapped in the vicious cycle of imbalance, it's time to seek help from a health expert.

Unnatural and nutrient-deficient foods, the pressures of modern life, and our polluted environment make it harder and harder for us to come even close to balance. I grew up in nature, surrounded by hills and rivers—that's where I thrive. When my husband and I first moved to New York City, it took me quite a while to adapt to the air, noisy traffic, lack of trees, and people rushing in all directions. How do I manage to keep my balance? The practice of yoga and Ayurveda works for me—and, yes, it's a work in progress.

What about you? What is *your* reference point for balance? How do you maintain it?

Balance runs on two tracks—avoiding the things that initiated disruption and perpetuate your imbalance and favoring the things that support your balance. This book is dedicated to helping you find your balance through diet, so as I introduce you to the concepts of food qualities and compatibility and eating with the seasons, keep in mind the universal law of nature: "Like increases like, and opposites balance." In each recipe chapter, I will guide you through creating specific balancing meals for the season, and each recipe will give you options to diminish the negative effects of Airy, Fiery, or Earthy digestion.

A NEW RELATIONSHIP WITH FOOD

QUALITIES OVER QUANTITY

In this chapter I want you to meet food and start the relationship anew. A relationship that gradually evolves and deepens as you understand each other's qualities, strengths, and weaknesses, and when or how you get along best.

But let's first go over your old ways with food. How many times have you tried counting your daily calories to lose or maintain your weight? How long did you last? Although keeping track of your calorie intake can be helpful for monitoring your food portions, it doesn't guarantee that you are eating the foods or nutrients that you actually need. We usually turn to the calorie calculator when we attempt to lose weight, but studies show that cutting calories can negatively affect our brainpower. Rather than limiting your diet by staying away from good fats, proteins, or carbs, it is better to eliminate "empty" calories coming from processed and artificial foods—these are the main culprits in weight gain anyway. Once you substitute real food for junk food, your body will intuitively regulate how much to eat. Just as in relationships with people, you want to be around those who help you grow and stay away from those who suck out your energy and give you troubles.

Throughout my life, I've never been overweight; all my health issues led to being underweight and even emaciated. I've never had to count my calories, but I still suffered from a long-term inflammatory disease, high blood sugar, and chronic fatigue. With the help of SV Ayurveda, I realized that eating the wrong foods in the wrong way was one of the causes.

Modern nutrition measures each ingredient according to its biochemical components and tells us how many calories or grams of protein, fat, and carbohydrate a food has and what vitamins and minerals it is rich in. These nutrition facts are helpful and necessary, but they only give us the quantitative information about a food's basic chemistry.

With Ayurveda, we can talk about food in the language of qualities that capture the food's physical and energetic properties. Instead of using measurements, we describe food according to how we experience it in our digestive system—what are the food's taste, texture, post-digestive effect, or healing benefits? That's how we connect with food anyway. You probably say, "I need something sweet," more often than "I need a few grams of sugar." Or, "Boy, this feels heavy in my stomach," rather than, "My stomach is filled with protein and starch."

With its unique qualities, every substance has some effect on the body and mind. To select the foods that are good for you, you need to understand their essential qualities. It doesn't have to be complicated. Simply consider your constitution, the strength of your digestion, and how you're feeling today and pick nutritious foods of opposing qualities to balance yourself. For example, if you have an Airy constitution and are feeling particularly airy at the moment—cold, light and ungrounded, and gassy, or you have dry skin—today you need foods that are a bit more warm, heavy, dense, and moist. Gradually, as you deepen your relationship with food, you will get attuned to tailoring your diet specifically to your needs.

The Five Main Properties of Food

Food properties fall into five main categories, depending on how we experience them in different parts of our digestive system. According to nature's law of polarities, every food, when taken in moderation, may benefit us with its attributes, or healing powers; when taken in excess it may turn into "poison" and cause challenges.

1. THE WAY FOOD TASTES

As soon as we put food in our mouth, our tongue judges the first impression: does it taste sweet, sour, salty, bitter, pungent, or astringent? Or does it taste off? That first impression is often followed by our facial expression, because taste governs the chemistry between the body and the mind. I bet your "sweet" face looks different from your "sour" face.

Every substance has its predominant taste, and each taste has specific physical as well as emotional effects on our well-being. The chart below gives you examples of foods for each taste. If you would like to learn more about the physiological and psychological effects of each taste, turn to the Appendix on page 249.

What does a balanced meal look like? Over the last few decades recommendations have changed: the USDA Food Pyramid rose and then crumbled to be replaced by the Nutrition Plate. I find the Ayurvedic guideline for a balanced meal much simpler (and probably more long-lasting): include every taste on your plate. The specific proportions of tastes depend on your individual needs and the season; I discuss this in the beginning of each recipe chapter.

Balancing the six tastes on your plate is the best way to keep your body and mind in top condition and to overcome food cravings.

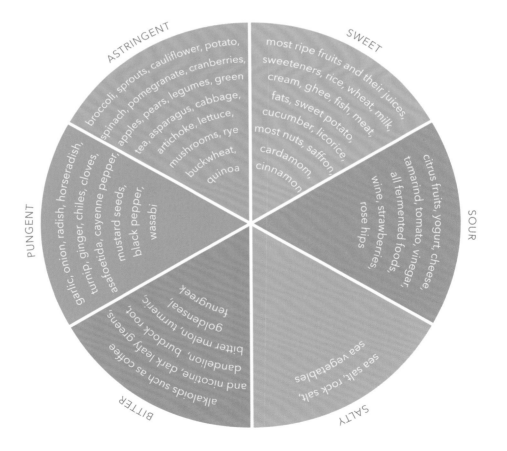

2. THE WAY FOOD FEELS

After the first burst of taste, subsequent bites reveal more about your food—its texture, temperature, and how it feels in your stomach. You're really getting to know each other, and you'd better pay attention to the "before and after" effect. When you eat something that tastes really good but later feels terrible in your stomach, your body is telling you that the food you just spent time with was not the best match. Your ideal food should be delicious and enjoyable at every stage of your interaction. In the introduction to each recipe chapter, I'll outline the best food matches for each season. Here are examples of the ten "gut-feeling" opposing qualities in food:

QUALITIES THAT PROMOTE STRENGTH AND GROWTH		QUALITIES THAT PROMOTE CLEANSING AND ELIMINATION	
Heavy	meat, fried foods, dairy, sweets, wheat	Light	puffed rice, popcorn, leafy greens
Dull	fats, meat	Sharp	very pungent substances
Cold	ice cream, chilled milk and drinks	Hot	ginger, chiles, garlic, alcohol
Oily/moist	butter, ghee, oils, avocado	Dry	barley, toast, nutrition bars, popcorn
Smooth	rice flour, all creamy substances	Rough	raw foods, dried dates, popcorn, chips
Solid	root vegetables, nuts, grains, meat	Liquid	all fluids—water, milk, juices, broths
Soft	banana, avocado, fig, butter, ghee	Hard	nuts, crackers, baked chickpeas
Stable	meat with bones, wheat, ghee	Moving	laxative foods, leafy vegetables
Bulky	meat, grains	Subtle	alcohol, tobacco, recreational drugs
Viscous	honey, gum resin, molasses	Clear	water-like, cleansing substances

3. THE WAY FOOD ACTS

Your interaction with food releases one of two kinds of energy: it heats you up or it cools you down.

Again, the heating and cooling actions are not determined by the thermometer but by the energy reaction after eating a food. A warm zucchini soup will have a cooling effect on your body, and cold tomato salad with garlic and chiles will heat you up.

HEATING (STIMULATING) FOODS	COOLING (CALMING) FOODS
chiles, mustard, flax seed/flax oil, onions, garlic, black pepper, honey, alcohol, saffron, sesame, lemon, wasabi	milk, cucumber, coconut, summer squash, coriander, fennel, melons, apples, pears, barley, aloe, almond milk, green beans, leafy greens

4. THE WAY FOOD TRANSFORMS

We are going much deeper with the transformation of food here: You had your first impression, you interacted and got to know each other, you absorbed its nourishment and let go of its wastes. Now we are talking about the deep transformative effect that the food has had on your body and mind. The concept of the effects of food after digestion and assimilation—how food transforms after it goes through the initial digestive process—is unique to Ayurveda. Modern nutrition tells us a lot about what the food is like before we eat it but not much about its subtle transformations. Knowing the three post-digestive effects of foods—sweet, pungent, and sour—lays the foundation of eating them in their proper combinations to ensure compatibility at every level of digestion. Specific examples follow in the next chapter.

5. THE WAY FOOD HEALS

Relationships come and go in life, but we remember people for who they are and what they are good at. It's the same with foods and herbs—we remember them for what they are good for. What remains after you digest the food, assimilate its nutrients, eliminate its wastes, and utilize its energy is the final memory of food, or its subtle action. When we talk about what a food or an herb is good for, we mean that special action that carries its ultimate healing intelligence. For example, cultures all over the world hold that pomegranate builds immunity, rose is good for the heart, and fennel regulates digestion.

So welcome to your new food world! The more you interact with and get to know an ingredient, the more you will know when to invite it to your plate and when to keep it on the shelf. Continue searching and you will find your "soul food": nourishing, satisfying, and supporting your optimal performance.

Understanding the qualities and nutritional content of food is essential for proper food compatibility, or making the best match for a meal.

Opposites That Don't Attract:
Learning to Mix and Match for Delicious, Digestible Meals

Imagine putting these people in a room together: an ambitious high achiever, a laid-back pacifist, a quiet daydreamer, a determined activist, and an unflinching pessimist. They may all be great people, but we can't assemble them and expect a quiet conversation.

It's the same with food. Every food is good for something, but sometimes eating two good foods together may result in them fighting in your stomach. Who suffers? You!

To enjoy a healthy relationship with food, you have to learn how to mix and match properly. Great chefs teach us how to match ingredients to layer friendly flavors and create stunning presentation, but if your goal is to make delicious food that you can digest without any problem, there are a few more key points to consider.

Following proper food combinations is especially important for the sick and weak and for those with chronic gut disorders. Mild digestive problems often result from eating conflicting foods and are easily solved by following the suggestions below.

- **Geographical location.** It is important to eat foods appropriate for the climate and altitude you live in. Certain recipes may be good to prepare in some parts of the world but not in others. Countries and cultures include specific foods to support the population in that particular environment, and people from other cultures and climates may not be able to handle the same diet.

For example, it would be incompatible to eat traditional South Indian (or any tropical) cuisine during winter in New York City. Or, even in freezing cold New York, it won't be suitable for us to follow the high-altitude diet of the Afghanistan nomads. The Mediterranean diet has proven to promote longevity locally, but does it work the same in other parts of the world?

- **Season.** It is contradictory to eat dry and cold foods in the winter and sharp and heating foods in the summer. Consult the recipe chapters to select seasonal foods.

- **Portion (depending on one's digestive strength).** Every person's digestive strength is unique. Depending on how strong your digestion is, you need to consider the quantity and heaviness of food you consume in one meal. If you have very strong digestion, you may eat big portions of heavy foods, but if your digestion is weak, eating smaller amounts and lighter foods would be best. For a person with weak digestion, it would be incompatible to eat food that is too heavy or oily or too much food in one meal.

- **Proportions in combining some foods.** Specific proportions of certain foods become toxic to the body. For example, equal parts by weight of honey and ghee (e.g., 1 teaspoon honey plus 3 teaspoons ghee) is toxic. So is the combination of equal parts of honey and lotus seed, and drinking very hot water right after eating honey.

- **Foods incompatible with one's work.** If a person of high metabolism performs heavy manual work or excessive exercise, it is incompatible to eat mostly Airy-type foods (dry, cold, rough, light).

- **Temperature shock.** In Ayurveda, we don't mix very cold and very hot foods, as it's not good for digestion or the health of your teeth. Your digestion will get confused if you have hot coffee or chocolate with ice cream, drink a glass of ice-cold water at the end of your meal, or drink cold fruit juice with hot tea or coffee.

- **Method of preparation.** Undercooked, overcooked, or in some cases food cooked without spices has a negative effect on digestion; microwaving kills the life in the food; heating honey makes it act as slow poison. These are just some examples.

- **Palatability.** There is no need to force yourself into eating supposedly healthy food while telling yourself "I hate this" with every bite—this alone will cause indigestion. It is much better to enjoy foods that evoke happiness and gratitude.

GOOD FOOD COMBINATIONS

Based on the concepts of the six tastes, food qualities, and digestion, the following foods commune well in a dish or a meal:

- **Grains** go well with all vegetables, milk, and yogurt.

- **Legumes** go well with grains (especially when cooked with digestive spices), non-starchy vegetables (such as broccoli, cabbage, cauliflower, radish, and asparagus), and leafy greens (such as kale, collards, chard, spinach, and lettuce).

- **Nuts and seeds** go well with milk, yogurt, leafy greens, citrus fruits, and sour fruits.

- **Starchy vegetables** (such as winter squash, potatoes, sweet potatoes, taro root) go well with leafy greens and non-starchy vegetables.

- **Meats** go well with light foods, such as non-starchy vegetables, leafy greens, and salads. Most of the common serving methods in

- Western society (steak and potato, chicken and bean burrito, spaghetti and meatballs, any meat sandwich, fried fish) are not optimal for digestion.

- **Milk** goes well with grains (such as wheat, rice, oats, amaranth, and quinoa), sweet dried fruit (such as dates, soaked raisins), ghee and butter, nuts, turmeric, ginger, pepper, cinnamon, cardamom, cloves, saffron, and vanilla.

- **Yogurt** goes well with grains, nuts and seeds, dried fruit (such as dates, raisins, figs, and apricots), non-leafy vegetables (such as summer squash, cauliflower, broccoli, radish), legumes, honey, and other sweeteners.

- **Cheese** goes well with non-starchy or green leafy vegetables, or may be eaten alone.

- **Raw fruits** are best eaten alone or in combination with other fruits of the same kind and same predominant taste. For example, it is okay to eat different berries together, or stone fruits and berries, or apples and pears. Fruit combined with nut milk is also acceptable. However, always eat melons alone because their high water content requires a very strong and focused fire to digest them. According to Shaka Vansiya Ayurveda, the only two raw fruits that commune with a meal at lunch are pineapple and papaya because of their high enzymatic properties. Cooked and dried fruits are an exception and suitable to mix with other foods.

BAD FOOD COMBINATIONS

The classical Ayurvedic texts give a long list of incompatible foods that could take days to study. Here I will list only the most common ones for us today—I've divided them into two groups: foods incompatible for slow (Earthy) digestion and combinations that lead to bad food chemistry and general indigestion.

Heavy Food Combinations to Avoid When You Experience Slow (Earthy) Digestion

- **Milk or heavy cream** with nightshades (potatoes, tomatoes, eggplant, and peppers) or eggs.

- **Yogurt** with nightshades or eggs.

- **Cheese** with nightshades, meat, bread, crackers, macaroni, beans, or eggs.

- **Meat, fish, or eggs** with dairy (milk, cream, yogurt, cheese), as they are very heavy and cause clogging of the circulatory channels in the body. Ayurveda completely supports the kosher concept of separating meat and milk!

Incompatible Food Combinations That Can Lead to General Indigestion

- **Milk or heavy cream** cause negative reactions when mixed with salt, sesame, or fresh fruit and foods of predominantly sour taste (such as fresh fruit, cheese, citrus, and tomatoes.

- **Yogurt** causes negative reactions when mixed with fresh fruit, milk, or leafy greens.

- **Cheese** causes negative reactions when mixed with raw fruit.

- **Raw fruit** causes negative reactions when mixed with dairy, cooked food, grains, legumes, salads, or leafy greens (see the above exception for pineapple and papaya).

- **Cucumber** does not go well with lemon because their prolonged "fight" in the stomach could lead to slowly accumulating toxins and calcification. Use cucumber with lime instead.

Resolving Cultural Culinary Confusion

There are many traditional recipes in different cultures of the world that call for mutually contradictory foods. If cheese and beans are a bad match, what do you make of Mexican cuisine? One way to resolve cultural culinary confusion is through the concept of homeostasis: our bodies are coded to do their best to maintain internal stability in order to survive, evolve, and thrive. They carry an intelligence that allows them to adjust and adapt in the face of challenging situations. If you repeatedly consume contradictory foods that do not cause an immediate reaction, your body will find ways to accept such a diet. However, it does come at a price. You may not experience discomfort right away, but in due course, depending on your body's weak points, eating mutually contradictory foods may result in deep imbalance. People in every culture mix incompatible foods, but we also see prominent diseases in every culture.

You can reduce the negative effects of bad food combinations with the help of spices. Spices enhance metabolism and act as connecting links between ingredients. Even in small doses, spices help reawaken our digestive intelligence. We'll learn more about spices on pages 227 to 233.

HOW TO TRANSITION TO EATING MORE COMPATIBLE FOODS

Food choices are very personal, and I understand that it may be difficult to accept the above suggestions at face value, especially after realizing that you may have been eating incompatible foods your whole life. The guidelines I share in this chapter are purely educational, offering an outlook on food from a digestion point of view; they are not meant to threaten or discourage anyone. The best evidence of what works for you is your personal experience. Some people are more sensitive and get an immediate reaction; others can eat anything without apparent discomfort. After years of not paying attention, I ended up with a bunch of allergies and an autoimmune disorder, and changing my habits to eating compatible foods helped me a great deal. I've seen too many allergies in children and adults who've eaten the typical American breakfast of processed cereal with cold milk, fruit, and orange juice for years. When we continuously give the body conflicting foods, at some point the immune system will sound an alert: "I can't handle this anymore!" and we develop allergies.

If you are open to improving an eating habit or two, I would strongly suggest you go slow. I've heard many wise people say that we shouldn't incorporate sudden, drastic changes if they make us unhappy. Life and eating are all about balance, and balance is the prerequisite to happiness. So, unless you are seriously ill, don't suddenly deprive yourself of your favorite incompatible dishes. That would reduce happiness, and being unhappy is definitely not balancing. Instead, begin to incorporate healthy changes in your diet by first trying a few of the simple suggestions for food combinations: for example, start eating fruit only by itself.

You can make food your best friend; you just have to get to know each other. Eating meals of compatible foods will help you to gradually restore your physiological balance and open and awaken your body's natural intelligence to heal itself. The more open and clean your body is, the less it will tolerate diets or routines that counter its innate wisdom and its alignment with nature.

General Meal Suggestions

IDEAL TIMING FOR BREAKFAST: 7 TO 9 A.M.

Keep it light but eat enough to satiate you until lunch. For most people, Cooked Apple Pre-Breakfast (page 143), followed by a cooked cereal or a warm smoothie, works really well. Meat and eggs could be too heavy for most people to fully break down in the morning, when digestion is still waking up.

IDEAL TIMING FOR LUNCH: 12 TO 1 P.M.

It is best to make lunch the largest meal of the day because digestion is strongest at midday, when the sun is at its peak. Favor a warm meal of cooked vegetables, lentils, grains, and heavy proteins with possible accompaniments of raw salads, desserts, and digestive aids such as chutneys and buttermilk lassi.

IDEAL TIMING FOR DINNER: 5:30 TO 6:30 P.M.

When the sun sets, so does our fire of digestion. The later dinner is served, the lighter your meal should be. Unless you have very fiery digestion, avoid heavy foods such as cheese, yogurt, large beans, meats, and oily and fried foods—they are too acidic for an evening meal and may cause acid reflux or prevent you from falling asleep on time. A lighter and smaller version of the food you cooked for lunch works too.

BEFORE BEDTIME: IDEALLY BY 10 P.M.

A warm cup of Calming Date Milkshake (page 183) or a soothing tea will prepare your nervous system for a sound sleep. If you have a flaring hunger that prevents you from falling asleep, try a small portion of food rich in protein.

SNACKS

Eat light snacks only if you are hungry between meals or if your meal is delayed. Fresh fruit, soaked nuts, and smoothies are good snack options.

Setting the Stage for Your Meals: It's Not Just What You Eat, But How You Eat It

You can have the healthiest, local, seasonal, organic, freshly picked, properly combined food on your table, but if you eat it at the wrong time, in the wrong way, or in the wrong quantity, ultimately that invigorating food will have some unhealthy consequences. Our digestive system is designed to absorb not only the chemical elements of the food, but also its subtle energies. A lot of us experience digestive problems because of unnatural eating habits. Long-term indigestion can lead to nutrient deficiencies and toxic buildup, which in turn can cause blockages, excess weight, unwanted deposits such as calcium in the joints or plaque in the arteries, or growths like cysts and tumors. According to Ayurveda, almost every physical illness can be traced back to indigestion. If you care about your health, do everything you can to maintain optimal digestion!

Here are some simple, enjoyable things you can do to support strong digestion, along with the possible consequences of the opposite behavior. Please upgrade your eating habits lovingly. Feeling guilty, being rigid with yourself, or enforcing healthy eating on those you dine with is not so healthy.

In my ashram years, I used to eat the yogic way: cross-legged on a cushion, in silence, with the fingers of my right hand (that's right, no cutlery!), then wash my hands, mouth, and feet after every meal. After lunch (not dinner), I would lie down on my left side and rest quietly for about twenty minutes. Today I am a busy businesswoman in New York City, and this yogic way of eating is not always possible for me, although I still enjoy it, especially when I'm at home.

EAT LIKE THIS	WHAT HAPPENS WHEN YOU DON'T
In a settled, harmonious environment free of distractions	Eating with noise, too many people, or too much movement around, or while watching TV, reading, or driving interrupts the brain-stomach communication, which disturbs digestion
In a peaceful state of mind	Eating when you're angry, upset, sad, or stressed out will only feed those negative emotions and cause them to flare up
In a sitting position	When you stand or walk, your energy concentrates on your feet, to support you, and thus weakens your digestive strength
Only when you are hungry	A lack of hunger means your digestive fire is slumbering and won't break down the food properly, thus potentially leading to fatigue, toxin buildup, and becoming overweight
At a moderate pace, neither too fast nor too slow, with thoughtful chewing	Devouring unchewed or partially chewed food puts extra pressure on the stomach
At an interval of two to four hours after a light meal, four to six hours after a full meal; this lets one meal be digested completely before the next (light snacks such as raw fruit or a few soaked nuts are okay)	Bingeing and eating heavy snacks between meals doesn't allow your digestive system to get a break and can lead to toxic buildup and obesity
Allowing at least two to three hours between your dinner and going to bed.	Going to bed right after eating is a recipe for toxicity, weight gain, and morning sluggishness
Without drinking a lot of water or ice-cold beverages. Drink water no less than thirty minutes before a meal and sixty to ninety minutes after a meal. It is okay to sip a little warm water or digestive tea with your meal, especially if your food is dry.	Drinking a large glass of water right before, during, or right after a meal tremendously suppresses your digestive fire
To only two-thirds to three-quarters of your capacity—a first burp is an indication to stop	Overeating leaves no room for the food in the stomach to move and break down properly and thus becomes one of the main causes of illness
At regular times	Eating at different times every day will negatively affect your body rhythms
With gratitude for the food you receive and praise for the cook	Eating without respect for the food or for those who prepared it sets up negativity and disconnection from nature and people—yet another cause for feeling unwell
Remaining seated for a few minutes after completing your meal	Rushing through a meal and jumping up from the table will feed your stressors more than your body

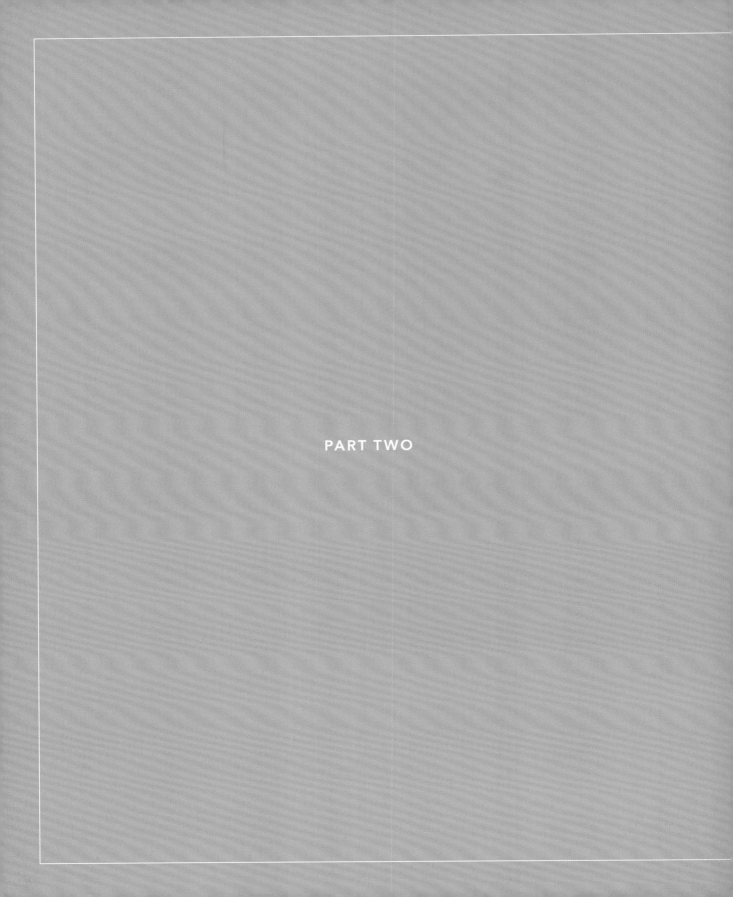

PART TWO

THE
RECIPES

About the Recipes

A lot of us today live in environments depleted of clean air and water, nutrient-rich soil, and peace and quiet. We become further depleted from excessive travel, work, family matters, worry, anxiety, and the hyperstimulation of our nervous systems through computers, video games, mass media, and too much entertainment. Now more than ever we need fresh, wholesome meals to balance the depleted environment and to stay strong in our life pursuits. That's why the recipes I have included in *What to Eat for How You Feel* are designed to nourish and calm us, down to the deepest levels of our being, in comforting and enjoyable ways. I hope you will experience the same satisfaction and inner peace that so many of my students and clients notice when they eat SV Ayurvedic meals.

Eating high-quality, wholesome foods is a core principle of health, but what is healthy for us at any particular time depends on our digestive strength, and our digestion is influenced by the changing cycles of nature. Seasonal changes can pose different challenges for different people depending on their constitution, imbalances, age, gender, and profession. Eating with the seasons is one way to live in the present, attuned with nature. Therefore I have organized the recipes to reflect our needs as seasons blend into each other and we enjoy foods from each of the three annual harvests in the Northern hemisphere. Seasons differ from region to region, and even that is affected by global climate changes. In fact, while writing this section, we celebrated Christmas in New York City at 72°F! That is why I also include seasonal ranges of temperature and humidity as guides—observe the temperature and humidity around you rather than just the months labeled on a calendar.

In spring and early summer when temperatures average from 40 to 65°F, we need energizing and cleansing foods to help us shake off winter sluggishness; in most cases, these recipes are also suitable for weight loss. In summer and early fall, when temperatures rise up to over 100°F, we need mostly cooling and hydrating foods. And in late fall-winter, when the lack of sun drops our thermometers below 65°F, we need warming and grounding foods to keep our balance. Just like we change our clothing seasonally, we also need to modify our diet. However, even when eating seasonally, we have to consider the strength of our digestion—that is the number one criteria for what foods are good for an individual.

For example, most people are prone to irregular Airy digestion in the middle of winter, but you may be experiencing the symptoms of Fiery digestion; in this case, when you are preparing a recipe from the Grounding chapter (for fall-winter), follow the variations for Fiery digestion. Whatever recipe you pick, consider my suggested adjustments to suit your digestion. At the end of each recipe chapter, I also offer menus for seasonal meals.

These are recipes I love and my students rave about, even years after they've been to class. Most recipes yield four servings; adjust portion sizes according to what else is included on the menu. Some recipes require a few minutes of advance planning such as soaking or making staples ahead. If some of my recipes look long, it is because I want to reduce your worries about whether you're doing things right by including detailed instructions; it doesn't mean they will take a long time. I believe that cooks (especially novices) deserve to know all potentially useful information to succeed.

What to Eat for How You Feel reflects my studies of SV Ayurveda, and although this ancient science originated in India, my recipes are not limited to the typical methods, seasonings, and appearance you'd associate with Indian food. With each recipe, I present a foundational principle of cooking for health and joy—by grasping the principles, you will have the freedom to adjust the details to suit your needs and taste buds.

Since some of the ingredients and methods I use are not yet common in Western cooking, I share knowledge in the recipe headnotes and sidebars intended to help you deepen your understanding of how different ingredients interact with and bring healing to our physiology. Take this information in bite-size pieces and let it unfold in your own cooking, feel it in your body, and let it eventually become your own kitchen wisdom. My goal is for you to discover the foods and recipes that open you up to your new ways of balance rather than confine you to rigid do's and don'ts.

All recipes are lacto-vegetarian and almost all of them have gluten-free and dairy-free options. I choose cultured ghee as the main cooking oil because of its high smoke point and numerous healing effects. Although derived from butter, ghee is lactose-free, so even if you are avoiding dairy in general, you might not react to ghee. If ghee is the only dairy-derived ingredient in a recipe, I designate that recipe as "dairy free" because I list vegan oil alternatives. The codes "GF" and "DF" indicate that the recipe is gluten and/or dairy free.

GENERAL SV AYURVEDIC COOKING GUIDELINES

Water: Pure alkaline spring water is charged with prana, and it supports the body's healing intelligence. Since cooking with spring water may not always be possible, opt for the next best: filtered tap water. Make sure to use pure water for soaking and in recipes that aren't cooked including beverages, sauces, and dressings.

Soaking: I recommend soaking for legumes, grains, nuts, and seeds to increase their digestibility and decrease their drying properties. Check the recipe you want to make in advance and plan for soaking ahead of time. It is best to rinse the ingredients until the water runs clear before soaking for the specified amount of time.

Toasting spices in oil: Most spices need heat to activate. When heating ghee or oil, start by heating a dry pan on low heat, then add the ghee, and when it is hot but not smoking, add spices in the succession the recipe recommends.

Making adjustments: The strength of basic condiments such as lime, ginger, chiles, and fresh herbs varies according to season and the part of the world you live in. Each one of us also has personal taste preferences. While following my recipes, you can always adjust the consistency and the amount of salt, sweeteners, and seasonings according to your taste and liking. Your palate is your best guide, so make your food pleasing to your senses. When you support your body with good food and restful sleep, your taste buds will sharpen their ability to send you signals about the foods you need. This is when your balanced body will communicate its needs through the tastes you crave.

SPECIAL NOTES ON KEY INGREDIENTS

Asafoetida: This resin resembles the sulfury flavor of onions and garlic and balances Airy or Earthy digestion; it is, however, too heating for when you're feeling Fiery. Although it is very difficult to find pure-quality asafoetida in the United States (the powdered version sold in Indian grocery stores is synthetic or adulterated, and most brands add wheat flour to it), I include it as optional ingredient in some of my recipes because adding a pinch of asafoetida will be much less heating and stimulating than an onion or a few garlic cloves. I use gluten-free asafoetida powder for all my recipes. If you are fortunate to find pure asafoetida resin, then use only two mustard seed–size crumbs for each ¼ teaspoon powder. See Sources (page 250) for purchasing options.

Baking powder: The best quality is double-acting aluminum-free baking powder. Avoid baking powder that is not labeled "aluminum free" to minimize traces of aluminum entering your system.

Black pepper: Always grind black pepper fresh, just before adding it to food, because ground pepper oxidizes quickly, thus increasing chances of acidic reaction in the stomach.

Cardamom (pods or seeds): In my recipes, I use green cardamom unless I specify black cardamom. Green and black cardamom have very different aromas—green cardamom is sweet and black cardamom is smoky—and they are not interchangeable.

Ginger: Use fresh ginger; I specify "dry ginger" or "sunthi" in the recipes calling for that option (see page 89 for an explanation on the three kinds of ginger).

Lime juice: It not only enhances flavor and adds sour taste to your meal, but it also supports digestion, which is why you will see it frequently in my recipes. It is important to garnish food with lime juice only after turning off the heat and letting the food cool down a bit, just before serving (food with lime or lemon juice becomes very acidic when reheated to the boiling point). Or instead of finishing your dish with lime juice, you can serve lime wedges on the side with your meal.

Rose water and dried rose petals or buds: These must be the edible type (*Rosa damascena*), ideally organically grown. Read the labels before purchasing. The roses you buy from the florist shop are perfect for beautifying your room, but they are not to be eaten!

Soma Salt: white Himalayan rock salt extracted from the mountains of North West India. Ayurvedic texts explain that in general salt heats the body, but Soma Salt is more cooling and therefore the best of all salts. It is a bit less salty than sea salt. Available at www.chandika.com.

Turmeric: I stick to dry turmeric powder. I explain why I do not use fresh turmeric root for cooking on page 231.

Creating a Balanced Family or Party Menu

Planning a balanced menu for your family or friends may seem complicated because everyone's physiology and combination of the five elements is unique. How do you meet each person's different needs at one table, with one meal? I face this dilemma almost every day, when mostly Airy me has to cook for my always Fiery husband or when I plan Ayurvedic meals for our catering clients.

It is easier than you think. Here are some tips that are simple enough to apply that don't even require familiarity with Ayurvedic concepts:

Make it seasonal. Eating with the seasons alone promotes balance. Check the introduction to each recipe chapter for ideas.

Include foods of all six tastes (sweet, sour, salty, pungent, bitter, astringent) with every meal. Using a variety of spices and other ingredients, you could have all six tastes in a single dish.

Plan for meal combinations of complementary yet contrasting elements. Combine heavy with light, complex with simple, robust flavor with something bland, a crisp texture with a soft texture (e.g. raw salad with creamy dressing).

Consider the colors on the plate. Not only will they make your offering beautiful and appetizing, but a colorful meal ensures a variety of nutrients.

Do not repeat vegetables and seasonings in different dishes. If you use a beet in your soup, do not add it to the salad or the sautéed vegetables. And don't put chiles in everything—many people cannot tolerate them in excess.

Start slow with new recipes. If you are introducing your newest recipe experiment to your meal, include some family favorites in the rest of the meal, just in case.

Make complementary side dishes and condiments to provide a prominent taste. I usually make the sauce or chutney pungent and keep the main dishes moderate or low on the chiles and ginger. In this way the Earthy or Airy who need extra heat can add a few extra servings of the sauce while the Fiery can still enjoy a full meal without discomfort. Check the introduction to each recipe chapter for ideas on digestive condiments you can serve on the side. For a party, I usually serve two types of drinks: one cooling (such as the Hydrating Drink, page 132, or Rose Tea, page 133) and one heating (such as the Ginger Mint Limeade, page 89 or Almond Milk Chai; page 181). Guests can easily determine if they need to warm up or cool down and appreciate the option to choose.

Spice up portions of a dish to meet your diners' needs. If you need to add extra ginger and chiles to satisfy the needs of an Earthy person while keeping others cool, then set aside a portion of the dish, toast the ginger and chiles in a little ghee or oil to crisp them, then add to the special portion. In this way you can increase the pungency of the dish without having to cook a separate dish.

Vary portions of each dish according to individual needs. For example, serve less grains, cheese, and dessert to those who're feeling Earthy and want to lose weight but more to those who're feeling too thin and Airy.

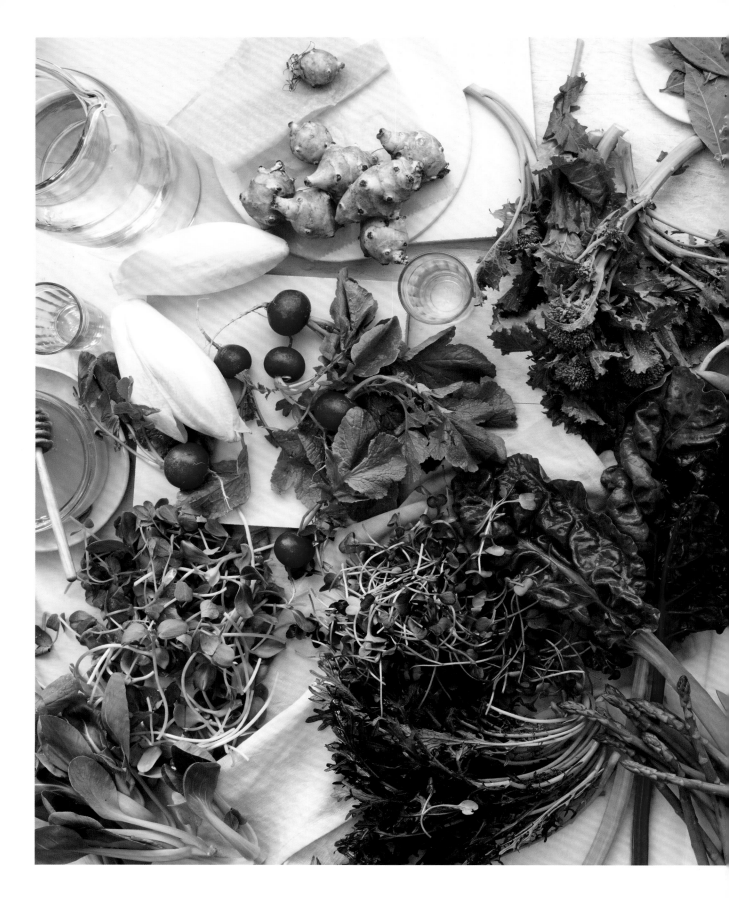

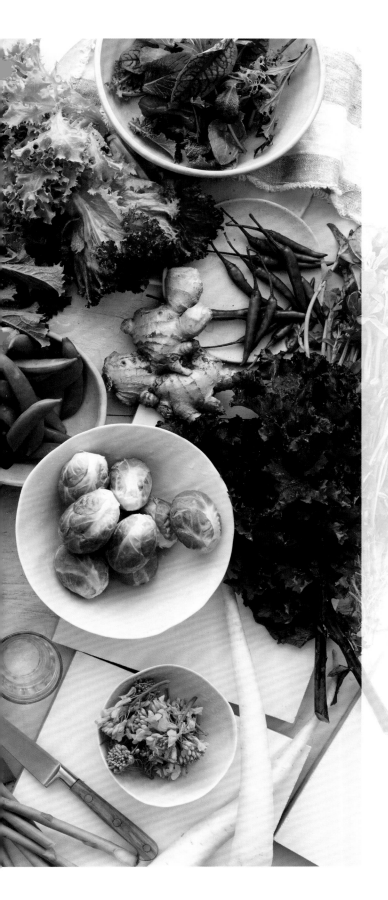

SPRING
&
EARLY
SUMMER

ENERGIZING RECIPES

Spring is a time for new beginnings and for releasing the stored energy we built in winter. It is a time for planting the seeds of health for the coming year.

Living in the northeast United States as I do, I always feel such relief at the end of a long winter. Finally the snow melts away, the air freshens up with the fragrance of moist soil, and trees and shrubs come back to life. With the warming temperatures, our bodies also begin to open up. Excessive mucus melts and rushes out of our system, and this is one reason why many of us experience colds and congestion in spring.

We balanced winter's cold and dryness with heavy, moist, sweet, fatty foods rich in protein. In spring we enter a new cycle with nature, where moisture and heaviness dominate the environment; therefore, we need to change our diet or our physiology will turn sluggish.

What happens to our digestion in spring? Due to the increased humidity in the atmosphere, we may experience a switch from Fiery or Airy to slow (Earthy) digestion, which means that an increased moisture in the stomach will lower our digestive fire and slow down our metabolism. Your appetite may go down and you may feel heavier and more tired than usual. That is why you need to gradually and comfortably adjust your diet to the balancing suggestions below. If you don't, perpetual slow digestion may lead to excess mucus, coughs, clammy skin, weight gain, and lethargy.

Spring weather temperatures usually stay in the range of 50°F and 80°F during the day. This is the best season for annual detoxification and cleansing because our microcirculatory channels naturally soften and expand, making the release of toxins much easier. Please keep in mind that before you indulge yourself in cleansing (and it must be the right practice for you!), you need to prepare your body, and especially your liver, by adjusting your diet and perhaps adding a few self-care treatments to your regimen. There is nothing more damaging to your system than a premature, harsh, or improper detox. In this chapter I have interspersed recipes that can be used during a gentle and safe cleansing protocol.

Balance with foods from the spring harvest: peas, leafy greens, dandelion, asparagus, radish, burdock root. We also need the dryness and astringency of lentils and small beans and the pungency of ginger, chiles, black pepper, cinnamon, cloves, ajwain, and cardamom. In general, favor warm foods that are dry, light, and predominantly pungent, bitter, and astringent tastes. Apples, pears, pomegranate, sunchokes, radicchio, broccoli rabe, cruciferous vegetables, and sprouts are all good spring foods. The drying properties of barley, quinoa, buckwheat, rye, millet, buckwheat noodles (soba), and corn make them perfect grains for spring. And get moving to enhance your metabolism—walk, exercise, hike, and dance more!

Stay away from foods that are heavy, oily, and cold and reduce the sweet, salty, and sour tastes in your menus. In this season you really want to cut down on sweets, nuts, wheat, brown rice, meat, dairy, avocados, coconuts, bananas, oranges, tomatoes, cucumbers, and sweet potatoes, because they may cause excessive congestion. (Although zucchini and lauki squash are watery summer vegetables, they support the cleansing of the liver; for that reason, I use them in small amounts in some of the recipes.) Raw honey is the best sweetener in this season (but avoid it if you have Fiery digestion). In general, on your plate you need less grains, more vegetables, and a moderate amount of light protein (preferably for lunch, not dinner). It is also good to reduce salt, which makes the body retain moisture. Avoid leftovers (especially refrigerated starchy foods), as their lower digestibility increases the possibility of congestion and weight gain. Refrain from napping during the day or sleeping after sunrise.

TIPS FOR IMPROVING SLOW (EARTHY) DIGESTION

Revisit "Setting the Stage for Your Meals: It's Not Just What You Eat, But How You Eat It" on pages 40-41—this practice is always useful, no matter what your digestion is. The following tips are specific for slow (Earthy) digestion; they also support natural weight loss.

- Follow the recipes and recommendations in this chapter.

- Chew 1 teaspoon of After-Meal Spice Blend for Slow (Earthy) Digestion (at right) after lunch and dinner.

- Eat three small meals at regular times (only when you're hungry).

- Drink warm water throughout the day.

- Drink up to 1 cup of Energizing Buttermilk (page 215) at lunchtime.

- If your appetite is low, before a meal chew 1 teaspoon minced fresh ginger sprinkled with a tiny pinch of rock salt (not sea salt) and a splash of lime juice.

- Cook with small amounts of sesame oil, black sesame oil (as a finishing oil), cultured ghee, and olive oil; avoid coconut oil.

- Follow a mono diet (eating only one thing all day) once or twice a week with Detox Kulthi Khichari (page 67) and Cilantro Chutney (page 191).

AFTER-MEAL SPICE BLEND FOR SLOW (EARTHY) DIGESTION

This simple digestive spice mix comes in very handy when you experience Earthy digestion and have to eat out a lot. You can conveniently carry it with you and use after meals.

Fennel cools off excess digestive acids and ajwain sharpens the digestive fire, ensuring that your food is properly digested and absorbed. If you are on a low-estrogen diet, substitute coriander seeds for the fennel. This digestive aid is also an effective natural mouth freshener!

2 tablespoons plus 2 teaspoons fennel seeds

½ teaspoon ajwain seeds

In a small heavy skillet, dry-toast the spices together over low heat until they darken a few shades and release their aroma. Remove from the pan and let them cool down completely, then store in an airtight jar. Chew ½ teaspoon after lunch and dinner.

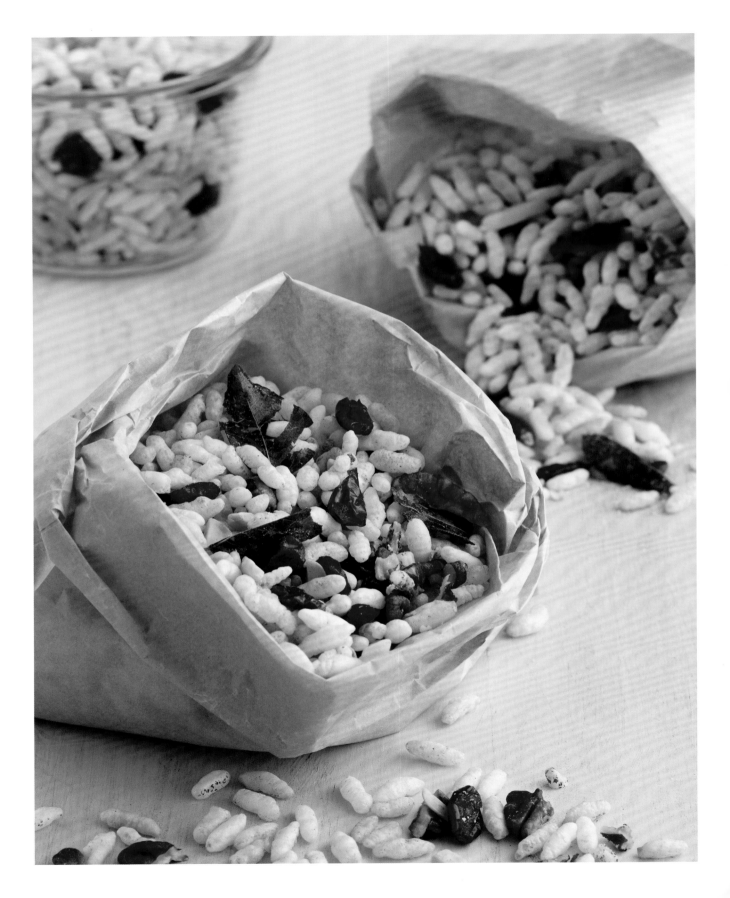

CRISPY PUFFED RICE

COOK: 5 MINUTES   serves 4 to 6 GF DF

Light, dry, crunchy—eat Crispy Puffed Rice for breakfast or munch on it as a light snack. It is a nourishing and tasty alternative to popcorn.

You can use any kind of puffed rice for this recipe, from the variety sold in Indian grocery stores to the different brands available in supermarkets and health food stores. White puffed rice is easier to digest.

1 tablespoon ghee or sesame oil

½ teaspoon black mustard seeds

6 curry leaves

1 green Thai chile, seeded and minced

½ teaspoon Energizing Masala (page 221)

½ teaspoon ground turmeric

¼ teaspoon salt

4 cups plain puffed rice

Small handful of chopped pistachios, pecans, walnuts, cashews, whole or slivered almonds (or any combination)

¼ cup dried cranberries

2 tablespoons raisins

FOR AIRY DIGESTION: Add an additional 2 teaspoons ghee in Step 1. Eat this snack occasionally.

FOR FIERY DIGESTION: Omit the black mustard seeds. Substitute Cooling Masala (page 221) for the Energizing Masala; omit the chile; replace the cranberries with more raisins.

1. In a wok or a sauté pan, heat the ghee over medium-high heat and add the mustard seeds. When the seeds begin to pop, add the curry leaves and chile and toast for a few seconds to crisp them; add the Energizing Masala, turmeric, salt, puffed rice, and nuts.

2. Stir-fry for 4 to 5 minutes, until the puffed rice absorbs the spices and becomes crispy; turn off the heat and add the dried cranberries and raisins. Mix well and serve warm or at room temperature.

3. Once the crispy rice cools down, store it in an airtight container, where it will keep for up to a week (it will lose its crispiness if it is not covered).

PINEAPPLE SMOOTHIE

SOAK: OVERNIGHT ▪ **PREP:** 5 TO 10 MINUTES   serves 2 (makes 16 ounces) GF DF

The pale green color and soft, slightly grainy consistency of Pineapple Smoothie make it a very appealing late morning or early afternoon snack. It is also a convenient and delightful refreshment to serve to between-meals guests. Just be prepared: the enzyme-rich pineapple will likely stir up people's appetite and make them hungry sooner than you think!

1 cup spring or filtered water

1½ cups peeled, cored, and diced pineapple

¼ cup soaked almonds, skins removed

1 tablespoon chopped fresh mint leaves

2 teaspoons maple syrup or sweetener of your choice (optional)

1 teaspoon grated fresh ginger

⅛ teaspoon vanilla extract

2 black peppercorns, crushed

FOR AIRY DIGESTION: Enjoy as it is.

FOR FIERY DIGESTION: Omit the black pepper and ginger.

Combine all the ingredients in a blender and blend until smooth. Add more water if you like. For optimal digestion, serve at room temperature. To store, refrigerate in a jar or closed container for up to 24 hours.

NOTE

▪ If you are pregnant, this smoothie is not for you, as pineapple can induce premature labor.

The Healing Benefits of Pineapple

▪ It is extremely nutritious, as it contains many essential vitamins and minerals such as vitamin C, thiamine, vitamin B6, manganese, potassium, magnesium, and even a little calcium and protein.

▪ It is an alkalizing food.

▪ Enhances digestion.

▪ It calms gastritis and overactive liver and acts as an anthelmintic (expels parasitic worms).

▪ Because it is an estrogenic food, it supports women's hormonal health by reducing hot flashes, stimulating breast milk production, and increasing scant menstrual flow.

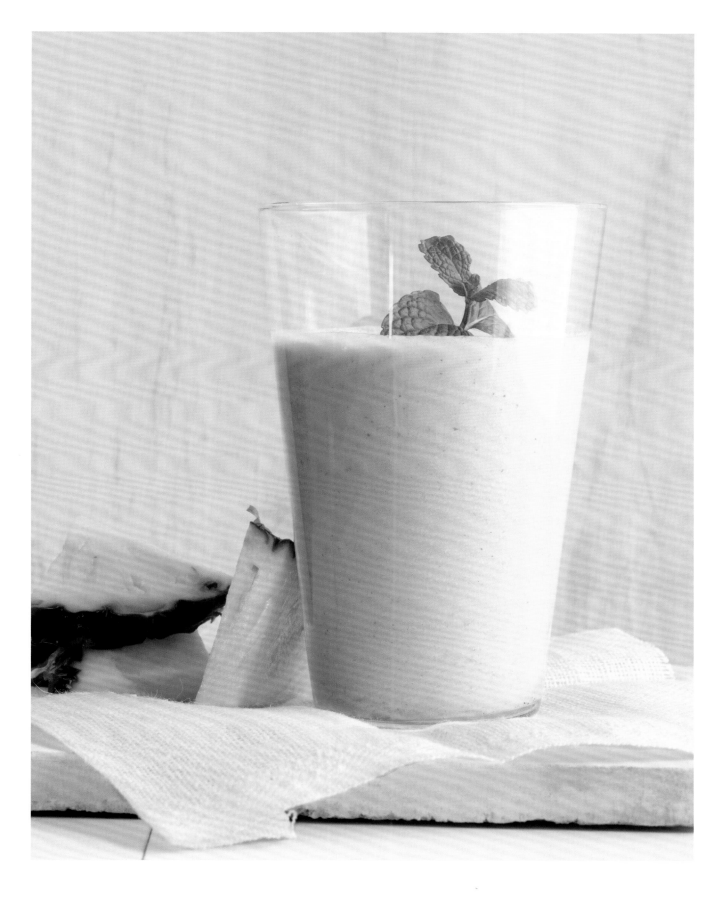

QUINOA FLAKES

COOK: 5 MINUTES

serves 1 GF DF

Time somehow seems to fly away in the morning, but that's no excuse to skip breakfast. This recipe is quick to make and quick to eat. It gives you a comforting full-but-light feeling and keeps you fueled until lunchtime. You could also make this cereal at night when you feel hungry but it is too late to eat a full meal. Quinoa flakes are available in health food stores and online.

½ teaspoon salt

½ teaspoon dried basil, Italian seasoning, or thyme

⅔ cup quinoa flakes

2 teaspoons olive oil

¼ teaspoon freshly ground black pepper

2 or 3 olives, pitted and chopped (optional)

½ toasted nori sheet, torn into 2-inch pieces (optional)

FOR AIRY DIGESTION: Add 1 teaspoon ghee in Step 1.

FOR FIERY DIGESTION: In Step 3, add 1 teaspoon ghee or coconut oil in addition to the olive oil and skip the black pepper and nori; serve with sticks of cucumber or celery.

1. Put 2 cups water in a small saucepan and bring it to a boil. Add the salt, dried herb, and quinoa flakes.

2. Stirring constantly, cook for about 1½ minutes, until the flakes have absorbed the water and are transformed into a creamy cereal.

3. Turn off the heat and add the olive oil, black pepper, and olives and nori, if using; cover for a minute to allow the flakes to firm up. As it cools, the cereal will thicken slightly. Add a little more water if you like a creamier consistency.

BARLEY AND QUINOA

SOAK: AT LEAST 1 HOUR ▪ **COOK:** ABOUT 40 MINUTES   serves 4 DF

Opposite qualities balance in this dish: the heavier, binding barley melds with the light, fluffy quinoa—both are very nourishing. Eating more of these grains in spring is very good, especially in preparation for detox.

Slightly sticky and chewy, Barley and Quinoa goes well with Pungent Lentil Soup (page 63), Broccoli Rabe and Cauliflower (page 70), and practically any legume or non-starchy vegetable dish. For optimal digestion, serve it with Cilantro Chutney (page 191).

½ cup pearled barley, soaked in hot water for at least 1 hour or overnight

1 teaspoon salt

2 teaspoons ghee or olive oil

1 teaspoon Digestive Masala (page 223)

1 tablespoon minced fresh dill (optional)

½ cup quinoa (any color)

FOR AIRY DIGESTION: Add 2 to 3 teaspoons extra ghee in Step 4.

FOR FIERY DIGESTION: Substitute Cooling Masala (page 221) or Superspice Masala (page 219) for the Digestive Masala in Step 4. Add more dill if you like.

1. Wash and drain the barley. In a small saucepan, combine the barley, salt, 1 teaspoon of the ghee, and 3 cups water and bring to a boil over high heat; cover, reduce the heat, and simmer for 15 minutes.

2. Soak the quinoa for the 15 minutes that the barley is cooking; wash well and drain.

3. Add the quinoa to the cooking barley; bring it to a full boil again, then cover and reduce the heat to maintain a simmer. Continue to cook until the barley and quinoa are soft and the water has evaporated, 15 to 20 minutes. If your grains are cooked but still a little watery, continue to cook them uncovered until the water disappears.

4. In a small metal measuring cup or a pan, lightly heat the remaining 1 teaspoon ghee, add the Digestive Masala, and gently stir for 5 to 10 seconds, until the spices release their aroma. Drizzle the spiced oil over the cooked grains, immediately cover the pot, and let the grains firm up for 5 minutes. Garnish with the dill and fluff with a large fork. Serve hot.

NOTES

▪ To make a large quantity, cook the two grains separately and fluff them together before Step 4.

▪ If you'd like to use hulled barley, soak it overnight and cook for about 45 minutes before adding the quinoa (a pressure cooker will save you time).

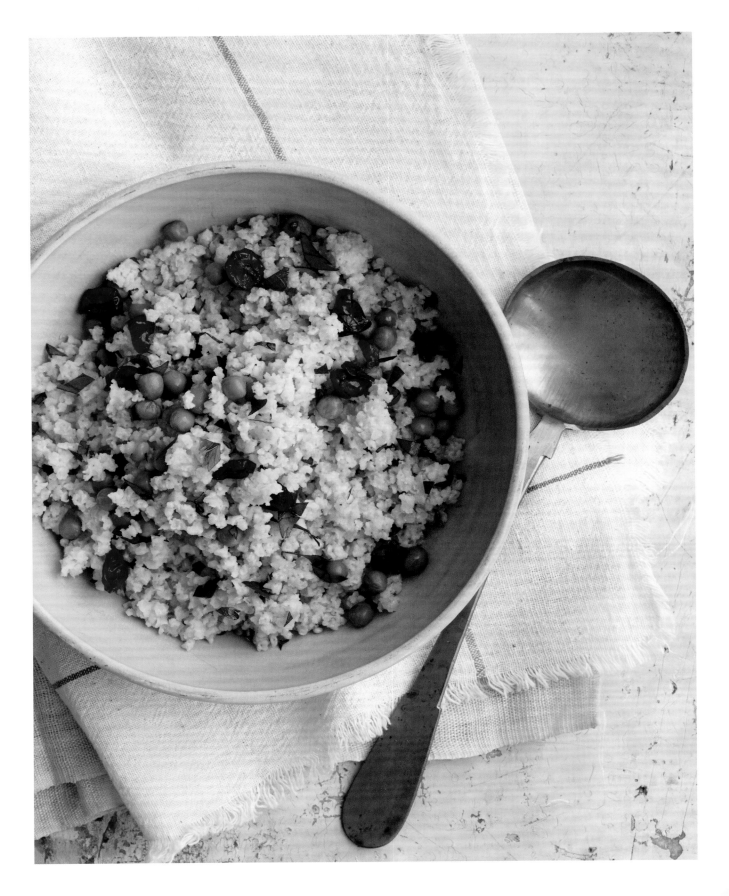

MILLET PILAF WITH
PEAS AND CRANBERRIES

COOK: ABOUT 30 MINUTES

With its light, drying, and heating qualities, millet is an ideal grain for when you're feeling Earthy. Because of its higher protein content, this tiny yellow grain takes longer to digest, but the seasonings I use in this recipe will help you enjoy millet without feeling heavy.

Millet turns rancid quickly, so it is best to purchase it in small quantities and store it refrigerated in a closed container.

With its mild, cornlike flavor and sweet-astringent taste, Millet with Peas and Cranberries goes well with Sunchoke and Asparagus Salad (page 77), Asparagus and Daikon Radish Soup (page 61), or Broccoli Rabe and Cauliflower (page 70).

½ cup millet (dry; do not rinse)

¾ teaspoon salt

2 cardamom pods, slightly crushed
open on one end

1 teaspoon Cooling Pungent Masala
(page 222)

½ teaspoon ground cumin

1 teaspoon ghee or olive oil

½ cup fresh or frozen petite peas

2 tablespoons dried cranberries

1 tablespoon minced fresh parsley, dill,
or cilantro

Splash of lime juice

FOR AIRY DIGESTION: Millet might be too drying for you, so eat it occasionally with a generous dab of ghee or olive oil.

FOR FIERY DIGESTION: Substitute raisins for the cranberries. Millet might be too drying and heating for you, so eat it occasionally.

1. To bring out millet's flavor, dry-toast it in a 1½-quart sauté pan over medium-low heat for 4 to 5 minutes, until the seeds release their aroma and darken a few shades.

2. While you're toasting the millet, bring 1½ cups water to a boil.

3. Pour the boiling water over the toasted millet and add the salt, cardamom, masala, cumin, and ghee and stir to mix. Cover, reduce the heat to low, and simmer for 25 minutes, or until the liquid has been absorbed and the grains are soft and fluffy. If some of the grains are still hard, add ¼ cup more hot water and continue to simmer for 5 to 10 minutes.

4. Turn off the heat and add the peas and cranberries. Cover immediately and let the grains rest for 5 minutes. Fluff with a fork and remove the cardamom pods.

5. Garnish with the fresh herb and lime juice. Serve hot.

VARIATION

- Substitute ¼ cup red quinoa (rinsed and drained) for ¼ cup of the millet; add it with the water in Step 3.

HERBED BUCKWHEAT

serves 4 GF DF

In Russia, buckwheat is what rice is in Asia and bread is in Europe—a daily staple. In the United States, hulled buckwheat groats are available as raw or roasted (kasha). In this recipe I use kasha for the sake of saving time and add herbs that support slow digestion. Herbed Buckwheat is quite filling; eat it on its own as a breakfast cereal or serve it as a grain dish with vegetables, salad, or soup. It goes well with Raisin-Cranberry Sauce (page 189) and Kale and Arugula Pesto (page 190).

1 teaspoon salt

1 cup roasted buckwheat (kasha), rinsed and drained (see Note)

1 teaspoon dried thyme or 1 tablespoon fresh thyme leaves

½ teaspoon dried basil or 2 teaspoons chopped fresh basil

1 bay leaf

1 teaspoon ghee, sesame oil, or olive oil

A few fresh mint or rosemary leaves (optional)

4 lime slices

FOR AIRY DIGESTION: Increase the ghee to 1 tablespoon. Cook with an additional ½ cup water to make the buckwheat moister. Buckwheat might be too drying for the Airy, so eat it only occasionally.

FOR FIERY DIGESTION: Substitute dill for the thyme and coconut oil for the ghee; omit the bay leaf; cook with an additional ½ cup water. Buckwheat might be too heating and drying for the Fiery, so eat it only occasionally and avoid it when you're feeling overheated or feverish.

1. Bring 2½ cups water to a boil in a small saucepan; add the salt, buckwheat, thyme, basil, bay leaf, and ghee. Cover with a tight-fitting lid, and once the water boils again, reduce the heat to low and simmer for 20 to 25 minutes, until the grains are soft and fluffy and the water is absorbed.

2. Pour into bowls and garnish with fresh mint, if using, and a splash of lime. Serve hot.

NOTE

- If you would like to use raw buckwheat groats, dry-toast them in a pan over medium heat until they change to a darker shade of brown before proceeding with the recipe.

The Healing Benefits of Buckwheat

With its astringent, sweet, and pungent tastes and heating and drying qualities, buckwheat is ideal to eat during the damp and cool weather in spring and when we need to reduce excessive earthiness in our body. Buckwheat is your friend when you want to get rid of congestion, high cholesterol, or unwanted weight. Technically a seed, buckwheat is gluten-free and also high in all eight essential amino acids, making it a good protein source.

ASPARAGUS AND DAIKON RADISH SOUP

PREP: 5 MINUTES ▪ COOK: 15 MINUTES

serves 4 **GF** **DF**

This simple and delicious soup is very good for the kidneys. Tender, light green, and unassuming, Asparagus and Daikon Radish Soup goes well with Barley and Quinoa (page 57) and Sprouted Mung Salad (page 78) or with Detox Kulthi Khichari (page 67).

1 cup peeled and diced daikon radish

1 medium taro root, peeled and diced (about ⅔ cup)

1 teaspoon grated fresh ginger

1 teaspoon ground coriander

¾ teaspoon salt, or to taste

½ teaspoon ground turmeric

¼ teaspoon freshly ground black pepper

1 teaspoon olive oil

1 bunch asparagus, fibrous stalk ends trimmed and spears cut into ½-inch pieces (about 3 cups)

GARNISHES

1 tablespoon chopped fresh cilantro or dill

3 or 4 lime slices

FOR AIRY DIGESTION: Enjoy as is or add an extra teaspoon olive oil.

FOR FIERY DIGESTION: Omit the ginger and black pepper; add an additional ½ teaspoon ground cumin.

1. In a 2-quart saucepan, combine 4 cups water, the daikon, taro, ginger, coriander, salt, turmeric, pepper, and olive oil. Bring to a boil over medium-high heat, then reduce the heat, cover, and simmer for 10 minutes. Add the asparagus and cook for 5 more minutes, or until all the vegetables are tender.

2. You may serve the soup hot and garnish with the cilantro and lime juice immediately, or let it sit uncovered to cool down a bit, then blend to a smooth or chunky consistency. In this case, reheat if necessary and garnish with the cilantro and lime juice.

The Healing Benefits of Asparagus

Astringent, sweet, cooling, and diuretic, asparagus is good for everyone. Although seasonal in spring, I like to include it in my diet at least once or twice a month throughout the year because of its many benefits:

▪ Encourages elimination of toxins via the urinary tract

▪ Reduces water retention

▪ Strengthens the immune system (asparagus is high in glutathione)

▪ Lowers cholesterol while detoxifying the body

▪ Reduces inflammation

▪ Helps the body deal with arthritis, rheumatism, and asthma

▪ May increase the success rate of chemotherapy

▪ Cleanses the kidneys and prevents kidney stones

▪ Antidote against X-rays and other forms of radiation

TOASTED PAPADAMS (BEAN-FLOUR WAFERS)

COOK: 10 TO 15 SECONDS FOR EACH PAPADAM   GF DF

Papadams, also known as papad and poppadum, are paper-thin, crisp, sun-dried wafers made from urad or mung bean flour. Indian grocery stores sell a few varieties. I prefer to buy the plain papadams, because the seasoned ones are often way too spicy. My favorite brand is Sanjeevani Organics because they are less salty and of superior quality than most. Indian restaurants typically deep-fry papadams in oils of suspicious quality, often reused. Toasting them on a griddle or open flame is much healthier and brings a papadam to its perfect crispiness in seconds.

Toasted Papadam is a fantastic low-calorie, gluten-free alternative to bread and a good digestive aid when you're experiencing symptoms of Earthy imbalance. Keep in mind that cooked papadams become limp as they sit and absorb moisture from the air, so make them right before serving any meal. You could also break up toasted papadams and use them as a topping for soups or munch on them on their own as a snack or as a sidekick to a dip or salsa.

Your choice of papadam, in the amount you desire (see Note)

FOR AIRY DIGESTION: Use the griddle method, but add 1 to 2 teaspoons ghee and pan-fry the papadams on both sides. Eat a papadam occasionally with moist foods to counteract its dryness.

FOR FIERY DIGESTION: Papadams might be too aggravating for you.

OPEN-FLAME METHOD
Turn a gas burner to medium-low. Hold a papadam with a pair of tongs just over the flame until the part nearest the flame begins to blister and turn lighter in color. This should take no more than 2 to 3 seconds. Set aside. Gently grab the papadam again, this time on the cooked side, and continue to toast by rotating and turning it from side to side until there are no raw spots left. Be careful not to burn it; if you do, discard it and try again—you will quickly get the hang of it. This method of cooking curls the papadam into unique shapes.

GRIDDLE METHOD
Heat a flat cast-iron griddle or pan over medium-high heat. Add a papadam and use a paper towel or kitchen towel to gently press and rotate it, allowing every inch to cook, blister, and become crispy. This method produces completely flat papadams and reduces the risk of burning. You just have to be careful not to burn yourself!

NOTE

- Torn papadams burn easily, so select whole pieces for toasting.

PUNGENT LENTIL SOUP

SOAK: AT LEAST 30 MINUTES ▪ **COOK:** ABOUT 40 MINUTES

serves 4 GF DF

The hot seasonings here are on a mission: to speed up metabolism, improve circulation, and burn semidigested sludge. Serve with a light grain, sautéed greens, and Cilantro Chutney (page 191) for an extra kick of pungency.

½ cup yellow split mung dal

½ cup red lentils

¾ teaspoon ground turmeric

2 black cardamom pods, slightly crushed open on one end

1 tablespoon grated fresh ginger

1 or 2 green Thai chiles, seeded and minced

1 teaspoon ground fennel

6 curry leaves

2 teaspoons sesame oil, ghee, or olive oil

1½ teaspoons salt

¼ teaspoon freshly ground black pepper

GARNISHES

2 tablespoons coarsely chopped fresh cilantro or dill, or minced parsley

2 teaspoons fresh lime juice

FOR AIRY DIGESTION: Reduce the ginger to 1 teaspoon, and omit or reduce the chile by half.

FOR FIERY DIGESTION: Reduce the turmeric to ½ teaspoon, omit the ginger or replace it with ½ teaspoon powdered sunthi ginger, and omit the green chile.

1. Soak the mung dal and red lentils together in a bowl with 3 cups water for at least 30 minutes or up to overnight, then drain, wash well, and drain again.

2. Combine the mung dal and lentils with 4 cups water in a heavy 2- to 3-quart saucepan. Bring to a full boil over high heat, stirring occasionally and removing any froth from the surface. Add the turmeric, black cardamom, ginger, chiles, ground fennel, curry leaves, and oil and mix well. Reduce the heat to medium-low, cover with a tight-fitting lid, and simmer gently until the mung dal and lentils are soft and fully cooked, 20 to 30 minutes, stirring occasionally to keep them from sticking to the bottom of the pan.

3. Turn off the heat and stir in the salt and pepper. Leave the soup uncovered to cool for 3 to 4 minutes and remove the black cardamom pods. Serve hot, garnished with the fresh herbs and lime juice.

NOTE

▪ You can try these add-ins (adjust salt to taste and water as needed): 1 to 2 cups diced vegetables such as asparagus, lauki squash, zucchini, daikon radish, carrots, cauliflower, broccoli, leafy greens.

VARIATION

▪ Substitute 2 cups sprouted mung beans (see page 78 on how to sprout mung beans) for both the lentils and yellow split mung.

MORINGA SOUP

PREP: 5 MINUTES ▪ **COOK:** 20 MINUTES

serves 4 `GF` `DF`

I am so pleased that scientific and health circles finally paid attention and stirred up a buzz around moringa. Known to Ayurvedic practitioners for thousands of years, moringa (*Moringa oleifera*) is one of the most nourishing and detoxifying plants on the planet. Most nutritionists recommend it as a super food but are unaware of moringa's powerful detoxifying properties. I first started using it when Dr. Marianne Teitelbaum put me on a cleansing protocol to conquer my autoimmune disorder. She told me that when cooking moringa, it is important to use binders such as taro root or arrowroot powder to ensure complete elimination of toxins.

The moringa tree is an integral part of the cultures of India, Asia, and Africa, and they can easily be cultivated in the subtropical regions of the United States. In many African countries, moringa trees are a solution to hunger. Although in the United States fresh moringa stalks or leaves are only available in Indian and Asian grocery stores (mostly in spring and summer) and are not known to Western chefs, I included this recipe in this book because of the dramatic improvements this easy broth can bring to your health.

Moringa Soup supports the cleansing of the liver, spleen, and blood, and by eating it regularly, it can gradually pull longstanding environmental toxins accumulated as deep as the bones, bone marrow, and nerves. It is best to sip this greenish broth for lunch, up to twice a week (daily consumption could overwhelm the liver).

Serve Moringa Soup for lunch with any meal but especially with khichari. If you cannot find fresh or frozen moringa locally, you can purchase excellent quality moringa leaf soup or tea powders at www.chandika.com. Other names for moringa are drumstick (in India, for the stalks), murungai, and munakkai.

4 fresh moringa stalks (8 ounces), chopped into 2-inch pieces, or 1 packet frozen stalks

3 medium taro roots, peeled and cut into ½-inch pieces (about 1 cup)

2 teaspoons Superspice Masala (page 219)

1¼ teaspoons salt

1 teaspoon olive oil

¼ teaspoon ground turmeric

1 small green Thai chile, seeded

6 curry leaves (optional)

GARNISHES

4 lime slices

¼ teaspoon freshly ground black pepper

FOR AIRY DIGESTION: Omit the chile; add a second teaspoon of olive oil.

FOR FIERY DIGESTION: Omit the black pepper and chile.

1. In a 2-quart saucepan, combine all the ingredients except the garnishes with 4 cups water. Bring to a boil over medium-high heat, then lower the heat, cover, and simmer for 20 minutes.

2. Leave the broth uncovered to cool it a bit, then transfer it to a blender or food processor and pulse 2 or 3 times (the goal is to finely crush the drumsticks, not puree them). Pour

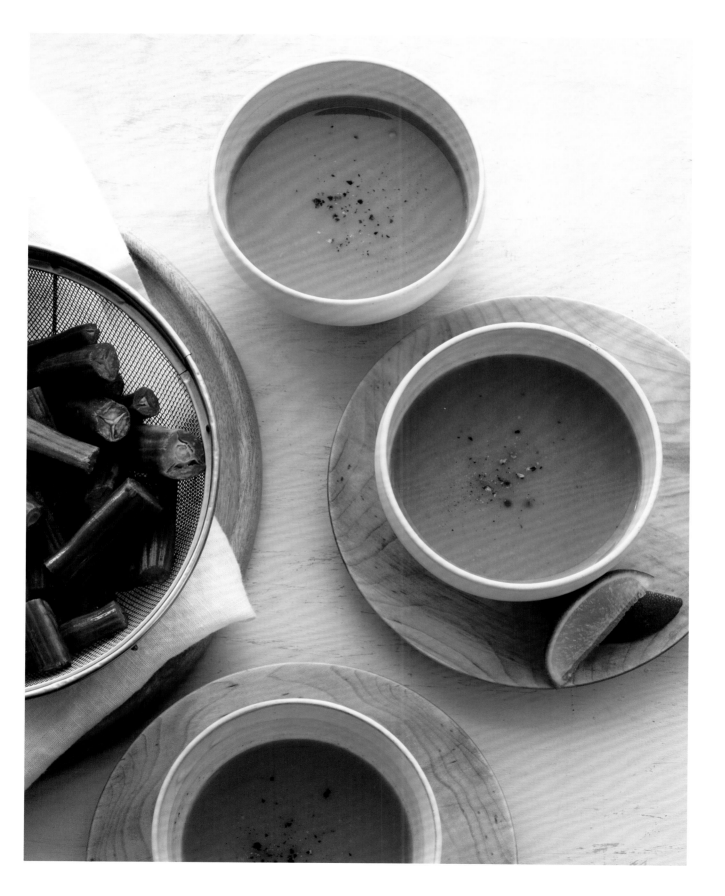

the broth over a mesh strainer with a pot
or bowl underneath and strain well, using a
spoon or your hands to press and extract as
much broth as possible. You will be left with a
bundle of straw-like moringa fibers—discard
them.

3. Serve the soup hot with a splash of lime
juice and a sprinkle of pepper.

VARIATIONS

- Substitute 2 tablespoons arrowroot powder for
  the taro root, adding it at the end (do not boil
  it with the other ingredients). Mix the arrowroot
  powder with 2 tablespoons cold water and add
  to the strained broth at the end of Step 2. Bring
  the broth back to a boil while stirring frequently
  to thicken it.

- Substitute 1 cup fresh moringa leaves for the
  stalks in Step 1. Cook for only for 7 minutes.
  Please note that moringa leaves are more potent
  detoxifiers than the stalks.

- If you are drinking this broth on a cleansing day,
  reduce the salt to ¼ teaspoon or omit it completely. Less salt in food helps switch the colon
  from absorption to elimination mode.

CAUTION

- Do not drink moringa juice (as promoted
  online)—it can cause liver detox crisis.

- Do not consume moringa during pregnancy (it
  could cause miscarriage).

- Because of its potent detoxifying action, it is
  best not to give moringa to babies. Infancy is
  primarily a time for nurturing and building, not
  detoxifying. Start introducing moringa to children of five years and older, when they can reap
  its nourishing benefits.

The Healing Benefits of Moringa

Astringent, bitter, pungent, light, and
heating—this is how the ancient Sanskrit
texts describe moringa. They referred to it
as *shigru*, which literally means "an arrow."
Like an arrow, moringa molecules travel
fast and penetrate deep into tissues of the
body, reaching all the way down to the
bone marrow. To compare its nutrients to
common foods, moringa has:

- Twenty-five times more iron than spinach

- Seven times more vitamin C than an
  orange

- Four times more calcium and twice as
  much protein as whole milk

- Triple the potassium of a banana

- Forty-seven different antioxidants

Some of moringa's medicinal benefits:

- Pulls toxins from the blood, muscle, fat,
  bone, bone marrow, liver, and spleen

- Strengthens the immune system

- Supports fat metabolism and weight loss

- Enhances digestion

- Increases fertility

- Detoxifies the skin

- Nourishes the eyes

- Reduces inflammation in the joints

- Lowers cholesterol

DETOX KULTHI KHICHARI (GRAIN AND LENTIL STEW) FOR WEIGHT LOSS

SOAK: AT LEAST 8 HOURS ■ **COOK:** ABOUT 45 MINUTES serves 3 to 4

No time to cook? Here is your meal in a pot! Pronounced KI-chah-REE and sometimes spelled *khichadi*, or *kitcheri*, in India the word describes any dish made with a grain and beans. We can safely say "as many cooks, as many khicharis," because you can prepare it in unlimited variations depending on the ingredients and cooking methods you choose.

Detox Kulthi Khichari for Weight Loss may not win an award for best-looking dish, but it is tasty and definitely a winner for breaking up kidney stones and relieving the body from impurities and excess fat. Even if you don't need to lose weight, you can make this recipe once or twice a month as a preventative, especially in fall and spring. Kulthi is a powerful cleanser, so do not eat this khichari more than twice a week unless you are being supervised by an Ayurvedic practitioner.

Kulthi beans are little known to most Western cooks, but they are extremely beneficial for detox and weight management. Sold in Indian grocery stores as horse gram (*Macrotyloma uniflorum*), these small brown beans have been used in Ayurvedic healing protocols for thousands of years.

¼ cup kulthi beans, sorted for bits of dirt or stones then soaked in hot water for at least 8 hours or overnight

¼ cup yellow split mung dal or red lentils, soaked in water to cover for at least 30 minutes or overnight

½ cup pearled barley or quinoa, soaked for at least 30 minutes or overnight

1½ teaspoons Energizing Masala (page 221)

½ teaspoon ground turmeric

6 curry leaves or 1 cassia leaf

1 or 2 green Thai chiles, seeded and minced

1 teaspoon sesame oil, ghee, or olive oil

1 medium taro root, peeled and cut into ½-inch cubes

⅓ cup chopped (½-inch cubes) peeled daikon radish

1 cup chopped (½-inch cubes) peeled lauki squash or zucchini

15 asparagus stems, fibrous stalk ends trimmed and spears chopped into 1-inch pieces

1 teaspoon salt

GARNISHES

2 tablespoons chopped fresh cilantro, basil, or dill

3 to 4 lime slices

FOR AIRY DIGESTION: Substitute white basmati rice for the barley and Digestive Masala (page 223) or Grounding Masala (page 222) for the Energizing Masala; the Thai chile is optional; increase the oil to 1 tablespoon.

FOR FIERY DIGESTION: Substitute Cooling Masala (page 221) or Superspice Masala (page 219) for the Energizing Masala; omit the chile; sesame oil is heating, so use ghee or olive oil for cooking.

(CONTINUED)

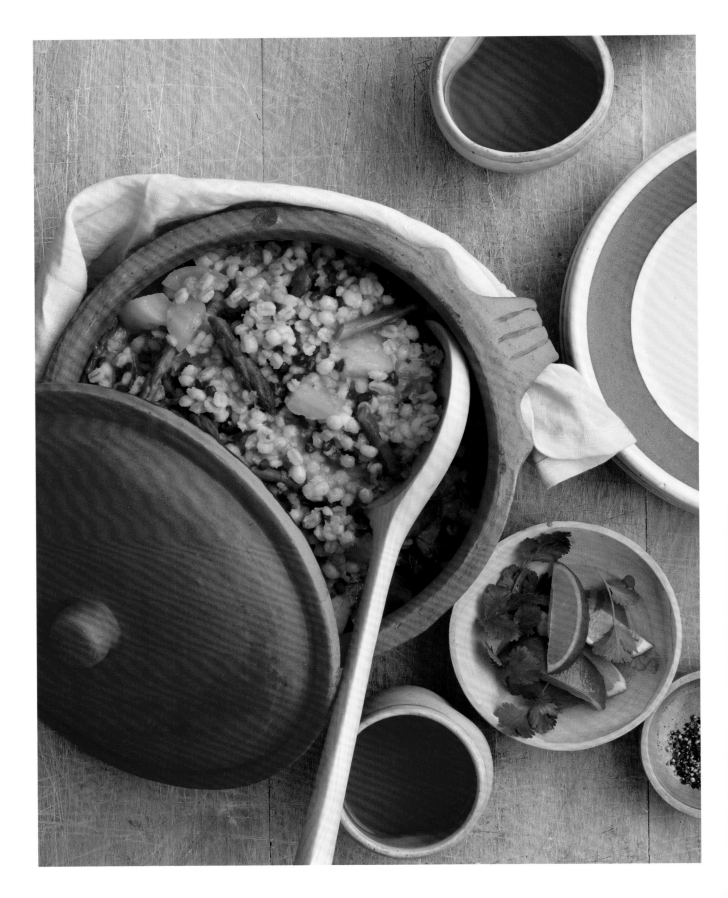

1. Rinse and drain the soaked kulthi beans. Place them in a blender with 1 cup water and blend until smooth. Rinse the soaked mung dal and barley together until the water runs clear.

2. In a medium saucepan, combine the kulthi beans, mung dal, barley, and 4 cups water and bring to a boil over medium-high heat. The pureed kulthi beans will produce a lot of froth—gently skim it off and discard it. Add the Energizing Masala, turmeric, curry leaves, chile, oil, taro, daikon, and squash, stir, then reduce the heat to medium-low, cover, and simmer for 25 to 30 minutes, until the mung dal, grains, and vegetables are tender; stir every 5 minutes to prevent the khichari from sticking to the bottom of the pot. Add the asparagus and salt and cook for 4 to 5 more minutes, until the asparagus is tender but still vibrant green.

3. Leave the pot of khichari uncovered to let it cool for 5 minutes. Garnish with fresh cilantro and lime juice and serve hot.

NOTES

- I use this combination of vegetables because of their cleansing properties. You could use 2 to 3 cups of just one of them or other vegetables such as broccoli, cabbage, kale, or Brussels sprouts, to name a few. You can also omit the vegetables altogether—if you do, use less salt to taste.

- Other ways of cooking kulthi: 1) Instead of puree-ing the soaked kulthi in the blender, you can cook the whole beans in 2 cups water with the lid on for 45 to 60 minutes, until soft, or cook them in a pressure cooker for 30 minutes. Combine the cooked kulthi with the rest of the ingredients in Step 2 and continue with the recipe. Although this method is more time-consuming, the khichari is less frothy and sticky and looks more appealing. 2) Toast dry (unsoaked) kulthi beans in a pan over low heat for about 5 minutes, until the beans darken a shade. Grind them to a powder, add ½ cup water, and pulse in the blender to create a paste. Proceed with Step 2. Use this method if you forget to soak the kulthi.

The Healing Benefits of Kulthi Beans

The classical texts of Ayurveda describe kulthi as mildly heating and astringent, light, and sharp, thus excellent for reducing excessive accumulation of the water and earth elements in the body. It has a very low glycemic index and is low in calories yet rich in nutrients including iron, molyb-denum, protein, and antioxidants. The main therapeutic value of kulthi is to decalcify, to break down and eliminate reactive toxins that have crystalized in the body. These are the very toxins that can cause gout if they wind up in our feet or hard bumpy arthritis nodules in our fingers, or they can harden our glands and arteries. Thus, kulthi sup-ports overall health by doing the following:

- Dissolving kidney stones and gallstones or calcium deposits in joints and arteries

- Burning fat, where toxins tend to linger

- Scraping and binding toxins for easy elimination

- Alleviating hemorrhoids

- Healing mild colic pains or ulcers

- Reducing water retention

- Strengthening the eyes

- Reducing insulin resistance

BROCCOLI RABE AND CAULIFLOWER

PREP: 5 TO 10 MINUTES ▪ **COOK:** ABOUT 20 MINUTES   serves 4 GF DF

Beautiful but bitter—how often do you encounter this combination? It may not be pleasant in human interactions, but it is definitely healthy in food. Broccoli rabe (pronounced "rob") is not really broccoli but rather a relative in the mustard greens family. It is beautiful yet so bitter it makes you squint; like most bitter foods, it cleanses the liver and reduces sugar cravings.

I added cauliflower to this recipe to buffer the bitterness of the rabe. Light, airy, and nutritious, this dish will help you shake off winter sluggishness and a few stubborn pounds. It is best digested at lunchtime.

2 teaspoons coriander seeds

½ teaspoon fennel seeds

½ teaspoon kalonji seeds

¼ teaspoon cumin seeds

1 tablespoon sesame oil, ghee, or olive oil

1 teaspoon minced green Thai chile

2 bay leaves

¾ teaspoon salt

1 small head cauliflower, chopped into ½-inch florets (about 3 cups)

1 small bunch broccoli rabe, stems trimmed and thinly sliced, leaves chopped into 1-inch strips (about 5 cups)

¼ teaspoon freshly ground black pepper

Fresh lime juice

FOR AIRY DIGESTION: With its lightness and bitterness, this dish will be challenging for you, so do not eat it often. Add an additional 1 tablespoon ghee; substitute 1 cup sliced carrots for 2 cups broccoli rabe, and cook them with the cauliflower; top with a grounding sauce, such as Sunflower-Sesame Dip (page 197).

FOR FIERY DIGESTION: Omit the chile.

1. Grind the coriander, fennel, kalonji, and cumin seeds to a powder in a spice grinder.

2. Heat a large skillet over medium-high heat. Add the oil, chile, and bay leaves and toast for about 10 seconds, then add the ground spices, salt, and cauliflower. Toss well, cover, and cook, stirring occasionally, for 5 to 7 minutes, until the florets look translucent and half-cooked. If the vegetables begin to brown and stick to the pan, add 1 tablespoon water. Fold in the broccoli rabe, cover, and continue to cook for 2 to 3 minutes, until the greens wilt. Toss and mix frequently until the broccoli rabe is soft yet still vibrant green and the cauliflower is tender and succulent, about 5 minutes.

3. Turn off the heat and sprinkle the vegetables with the pepper and lime. Serve hot.

VARIATION

▪ Substitute kale, collards, or other greens for the broccoli rabe.

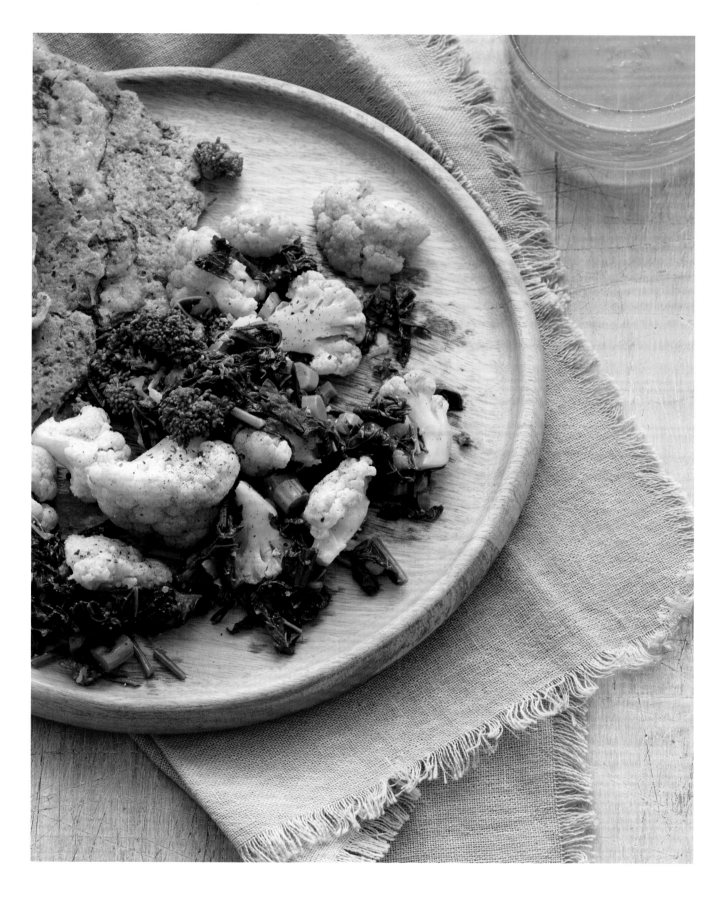

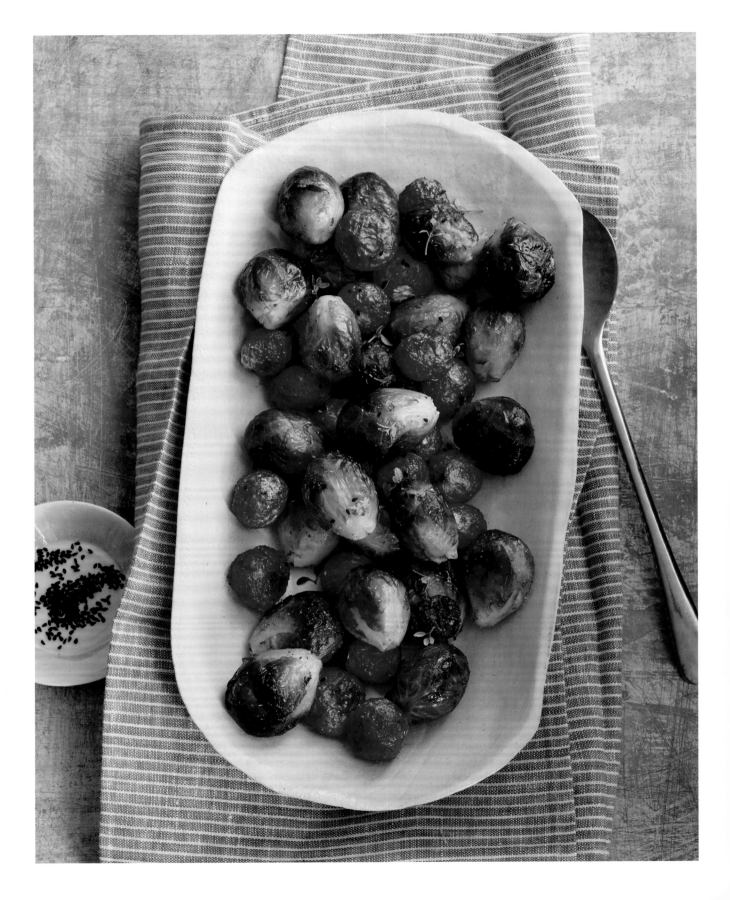

ROASTED BRUSSELS SPROUTS AND RED RADISHES

PREP: 10 MINUTES ▪ **COOK:** ABOUT 35 MINUTES   serves 4 `GF` `DF`

Brussels sprouts are one of those compelling vegetables: you either love them or hate them. With their bitter, pungent, and sweet tastes and heating qualities, Brussels sprouts and red radishes are ideal for busting sluggishness in late winter and early spring weather. Cooking those mini cabbages well neutralizes their bitterness and strong sulfury flavor. Select smaller Brussels sprouts, ideally attached to their growing stalk.

The sweet-pungent-bitter taste of these tender, ball-like vegetables will happily bounce on your palate. For a balancing energizing meal, serve Roasted Brussels Sprouts with Herbed Buckwheat (page 60) or Millet Pilaf with Peas and Cranberries (page 59) and a drizzle of Pink Tahini Dressing (page 199).

1½ teaspoons salt

4 cups (1 pound) Brussels sprouts (preferably smaller size), washed, stem ends trimmed, and an X cut into the base of each piece

2 cups small red radishes, ends trimmed

1 tablespoon melted ghee or sesame oil

1 teaspoon ground coriander

1 tablespoon grated fresh ginger

¼ teaspoon ground nutmeg

GARNISHES

1 teaspoon fresh thyme leaves

1 tablespoon fresh orange juice, or to taste

1 teaspoon fresh lime juice

A few turns of the peppermill

½ teaspoon toasted kalonji seeds

Pink Tahini Dressing (page 199)

FOR AIRY DIGESTION: This dish might be too aggravating for you if you're feeling very Airy. If you want to give it a try, add a teaspoon or two more ghee during roasting and 2 tablespoons lightly roasted walnuts in Step 3.

FOR FIERY DIGESTION: Brussels sprouts might be too heating for you. Replace them with green or red cabbage. Reduce the ginger to 1 teaspoon.

1. Preheat the oven to 400°F (350°F if using sesame oil).

2. Bring 6 cups of water with 1 teaspoon salt to a rolling boil in a large pot. Add the Brussels sprouts and cook until crisp-tender, about 6 minutes. Drain.

3. Lay the Brussels sprouts and radishes in a baking dish (a 9 x 13-inch Pyrex pan works well). Top with the ghee, coriander, ginger, the remaining ½ teaspoon salt, and the nutmeg and mix well. Level the vegetables on the dish. Roast for 25 to 30 minutes, until the vegetables are golden and crusty.

(CONTINUED)

4. Remove from the oven, transfer the vegetables to a serving dish, and let them cool down a bit, then garnish them with thyme, orange and lime juice, pepper, and toasted kalonji seeds. Serve immediately with a drizzle of Pink Tahini Dressing.

NOTES

- If your Brussels sprouts are larger than 1 inch, cut them in half or quarters.

- If you are planning to reheat this dish later, reserve the garnishes and add them just before serving.

The Healing Benefits of Brussels Sprouts

This petite cousin of cabbage is medicinal in many ways:

- Excellent source of folic acid, vitamins C and K, beta-carotene, and potassium

- Support the functions of the stomach and large intestine

- Gently stimulate the liver out of stagnancy

- Contain numerous cancer-fighting phytochemicals

- Bind mercury molecules (from the sulfur); when cooked with coriander and cilantro, Brussels sprouts help eliminate mercury from the body

GREEN CABBAGE AND KALE

PREP: 5 MINUTES ▪ **COOK:** ABOUT 15 MINUTES

serves 4 `GF` `DF`

This recipe makes cabbage enjoyable. Some people (especially the Airy) avoid cruciferous vegetables like cabbage and kale because of the gassy consequences. However, when cooked in the right way with heating spices (as in this recipe), your airs should remain contained. With its vibrant green colors, succulent yet chewy texture, and enticing aroma, this dish is a winner when you need to lighten up or have just twenty minutes to whip up a meal. It goes well with grains, fresh cheese, chutneys, soups, and breads.

1 tablespoon ghee or sesame oil

1 tablespoon olive oil

½ teaspoon kalonji seeds or cumin seeds

1 teaspoon grated fresh ginger

1 green Thai chile, seeded and minced

¼ teaspoon freshly ground black pepper

⅛ teaspoon asafoetida (optional)

4 cups chopped (½-inch strips) green cabbage

4 cups stemmed and torn or chopped (2-inch pieces) kale (any kind)

¾ teaspoon salt

Sprinkle of fresh lime juice

FOR AIRY DIGESTION: Omit the green chile; add 1 cup Golden Cheese Cubes (page 193) along with the kale in Step 2.

FOR FIERY DIGESTION: Omit the green chile and asafoetida (and black pepper if you have acidic stomach); add 1 cup Golden Cheese Cubes (page 193) along with the kale in Step 2.

1. In a large skillet, heat the ghee and olive oil over medium-low heat until hot but not smoking. Add the kalonji seeds and cook for about 10 seconds, then add the ginger, chile, black pepper, and asafoetida, if using. Immediately stir in the cabbage and 3 tablespoons water.

Cover and continue to cook over medium-low heat for at least 10 minutes, until the cabbage is soft and translucent. If the cabbage looks dry and is starting to stick to the bottom of the pan, add a little more water to prevent burning.

2. Fold in the kale and cover for a minute to let the kale wilt. Stir well and cook uncovered until the kale is soft but still vibrant green. Turn off the heat and add the salt and lime juice. Your vegetables should be succulent but without excess liquid in the pan.

The Healing Benefits of Cabbage

Cabbage and kale are botanical cousins. Humble yet powerful, cabbage is one of the least expensive vitamin-protective foods and one of the most healthful vegetables. It is an excellent source of vitamin C and a fair source of vitamins A, B1, and riboflavin. It is an alkaline food with a very low calorie content, which is why it is perfect for helping the Earthy lose weight. Cabbage is also rich in minerals: calcium, potassium, chlorine, iodine, phosphorus, sodium, and sulfur.

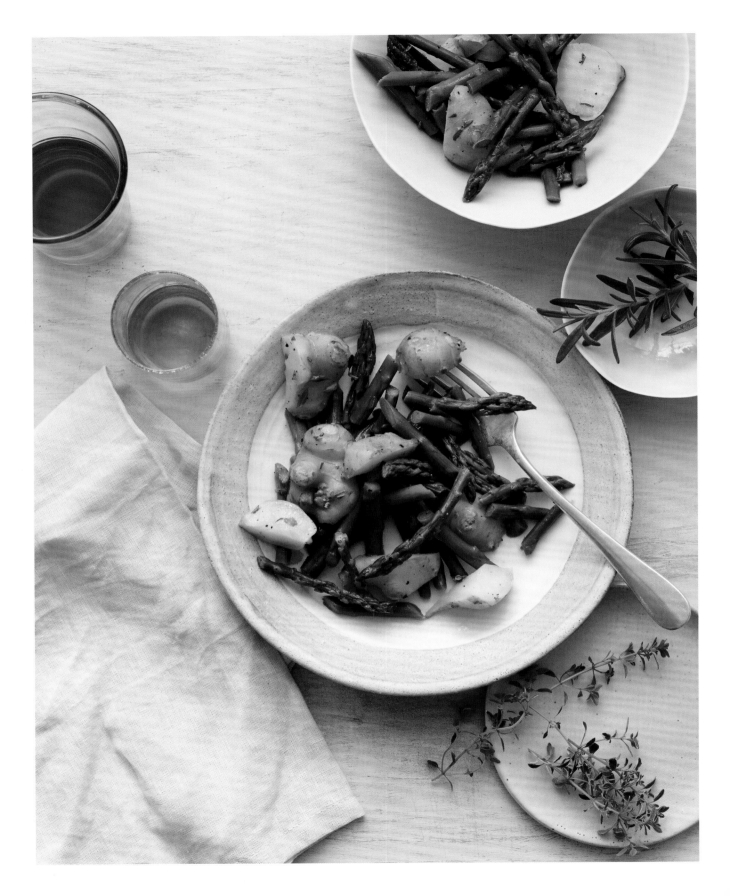

SUNCHOKE AND ASPARAGUS SALAD

PREP: 5 MINUTES ▪ COOK: 15 MINUTES

serves 4 GF DF

The sunchoke, also known as Jerusalem artichoke, has an astringent-sweet taste with delicate, almost artichoke-like flavor, which I find very pleasant and refreshing. Although you can eat sunchokes raw, I highly recommend lightly cooking them to reduce their exuberant airy qualities. Peeling these tubers is preferred but more time-consuming (and patience-testing); scrub them well with a vegetable brush when you're cooking them in a hurry.

2 cups scrubbed and chopped (1½-inch pieces) sunchokes (about 12 ounces)

1 bunch asparagus, fibrous stalk ends trimmed and spears cut into 2-inch pieces (about 2 cups)

DRESSING

1 teaspoon black sesame oil or olive oil

1 tablespoon fresh lime juice

1 tablespoon ginger juice (see Note)

1 teaspoon fresh thyme leaves or ¼ teaspoon dried thyme

½ teaspoon salt

½ teaspoon finely minced fresh rosemary leaves

¼ teaspoon freshly ground black pepper

¼ teaspoon ground nutmeg

FOR AIRY DIGESTION: Increase the oil to 1 tablespoon and omit the nutmeg; substitute parsnips for the sunchokes.

FOR FIERY DIGESTION: Omit the ginger juice and increase the oil to 1 tablespoon.

1. Steam the sunchokes in a steamer basket set over a pan of simmering water for about 10 minutes, until they are crisp-tender; remove from the steamer to a serving dish and set aside. Steam the asparagus for about 5 minutes, until tender, and plunge it in cold water to refresh it; drain well. Add to the dish with the sunchokes.

2. Whisk all the dressing ingredients in a small bowl, pour over the vegetables, and let them marinate for 5 to 10 minutes. Serve at room temperature.

NOTE

▪ To make ginger juice: Grate a 2-inch piece of ginger and squeeze the juice from it in your hand.

The Healing Benefits of Sunchokes

Unlike most root vegetables, sunchokes do not have starchy carbohydrates.

▪ Good source of inulin (a natural fructose that is medicinal for diabetics)

▪ Nourish the lungs

▪ Support the liver

▪ Treat constipation

▪ Aphrodisiac

▪ Good source of iron, potassium, and phosphorus

SPROUTED MUNG SALAD

SOAK AND SPROUT: AT LEAST 8 HOURS SOAKING; 4 TO 6 HOURS SPROUTING, DEPENDING ON ROOM TEMPERATURE ▪ **COOK AND COOL:** 15 MINUTES

serves 4 GF DF

Sprouted mung beans remind me of the precious time I spent with Yamuna Devi, one of my cooking mentors and author of two award-winning cookbooks. While showing me a dish with mung sprouts, she explained that the shoots have to be just budding. The longer the shoots are, the more starchy and sweet the beans will be. Budding shoots retain the predominant astringent taste and crunchiness of the beans.

Many nutritionists recommend sprouting beans, seeds, and grains as a way to increase nutritional value, digestibility, and prana. However, Ayurveda warns us that sprouting also increases Airy energy in the food, and raw sprouts can make you very spacy and gassy. Lightly sautéing the sprouts infuses them with more grounding and Fiery energy while retaining most of the nutrients.

½ cup whole mung beans (organic mung beans sprout best)

1 teaspoon sesame oil or olive oil

1 teaspoon black sesame seeds

1 tablespoon thinly julienned fresh ginger

1 green Thai chile, seeded and minced

¾ teaspoon salt

⅛ teaspoon asafoetida (optional)

¼ teaspoon freshly ground black pepper

3 cups packed baby arugula or watercress, rinsed and drained

½ cup sliced red radishes

2 tablespoons chopped fresh basil leaves

1 tablespoon fresh lime juice, or to taste

FOR AIRY DIGESTION: Increase the oil to 1 tablespoon and cook the sprouts with 2 tablespoons water for 5 more minutes. Add 1 tablespoon chopped walnuts and half a sliced avocado for more grounding at the end of recipe, just before serving.

FOR FIERY DIGESTION: Omit the asafoetida, black pepper, and chile; reduce the ginger to 1 teaspoon or replace it with ½ teaspoon powdered sunthi ginger (see page 89).

TO SPROUT THE MUNG BEANS

1. In a medium bowl, cover the mung beans with 2 cups cold water and let them soak at room temperature for at least 8 hours or overnight. Drain and rinse the mung beans.

2. There are a number of ways to sprout the soaked beans: If you have a special sprouting device such as a jar, bag, or plastic sprouter, follow the instructions of the manufacturer. Another way to sprout is to spread the beans in a mesh strainer or colander atop a bowl and cover the strainer with a lid or towel; keep in a dark corner of your kitchen. Splash the sprouts with water every couple of hours to maintain their moisture until they grow small shoots, no longer than ⅛ inch, about 4 to 6 hours. If you are not ready to use your fresh sprouts, you can cover and refrigerate them for up to 3 days. Always rinse and drain the sprouts before cooking them.

(CONTINUED)

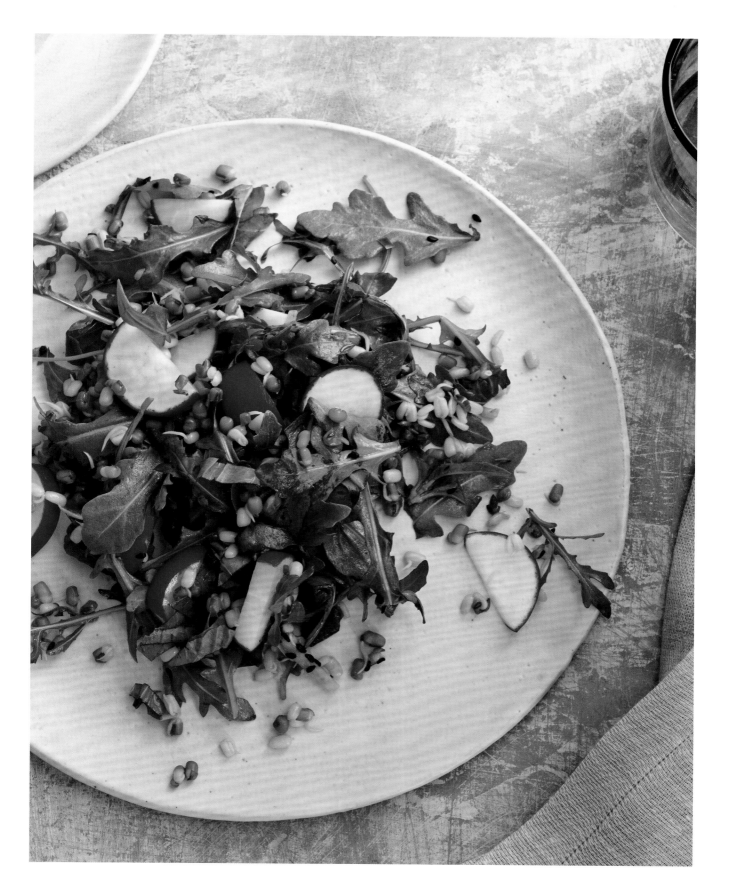

TO MAKE THE SALAD

1. In a medium sauté pan, heat the oil over medium-low heat. Add the black sesame seeds, ginger, and chile and toast for 10 seconds, then add the salt, asafoetida, if using, the black pepper, and mung sprouts. Sauté for 5 to 10 minutes, until the sprouts absorb the spiced oil and soften. Add the arugula and give it a few turns so it can mix with the sprouts and soften.

2. Turn off the heat and let the mung sprouts cool to room temperature. Toss in the sliced radishes, basil, and lime juice. Serve immediately.

The Healing Benefits of Mung

According to the ancient Ayurvedic texts, mung beans are the best of all legumes. They are easy to digest, with an astringent-sweet taste and cooling energy, and they are a good source of vegetable protein and fiber. When cooked or eaten with rice or other partial-protein grains, they provide the body with complete vegetable protein. They are slightly detoxifying, as they clean the gut of undigested food residue. Mung beans alleviate the challenges of the Fiery and the Earthy. Because they may slightly aggravate the Airy, mung beans need to be cooked with the appropriate spices and condiments, as in this recipe.

SKILLET VEGETABLE PIE (OR PANCAKES)

SOAK: OVERNIGHT ■ **PREP:** 10 MINUTES ■
COOK: ABOUT 35 MINUTES

makes one 10-inch pie or about 8 pancakes `GF` `DF`

Once I was invited to serve brunch to Deepak Chopra at his home in New York City. I made him this recipe as vegetable pancakes with Cilantro Chutney. I hope you will enjoy and rave about these pancakes as much as Deepak Chopra did!

Depending on how much time and energy you have, you can cook the batter as a low-maintenance rustic vegetable pie or as more labor-intensive but somewhat more refined crepe-like pancakes. The result is equally delicious and colorful—like a painter's palette—with its smudged spread of purple, green, orange, and yellow colors. I love this dish because it is free from gluten, very nutritious, and at the same time light and satisfying. Serve the pie or pancakes warm for a special breakfast, brunch, or side dish at lunch or dinner. It is also a great travel food. Whether you're flying or hiking, take a few slices of Vegetable Pie with you to munch on as you gaze at the clear sky.

Many thanks to my friend Kandarpa Bhuckory for the inspiration to create this recipe. It goes well with Cilantro Chutney (page 191) or Raisin-Cranberry Sauce (page 189).

1 cup yellow split mung dal, soaked overnight and drained

1 cup water

1 tablespoon grated fresh ginger

1 small green Thai chile, seeded and minced

1 tablespoon fresh lime juice

1½ teaspoons Digestive Masala (page 223)

1¼ teaspoons salt

½ teaspoon ground turmeric

⅛ teaspoon asafoetida (optional)

½ cup grated carrots

½ cup grated zucchini

½ cup grated red cabbage

1 cup packed (cut into ⅛-inch thin ribbons) spinach

1 tablespoon chopped fresh cilantro

1 tablespoon chopped fresh mint

Ghee or coconut oil, for cooking

FOR AIRY DIGESTION: This recipe is perfectly balancing for you. You could brush the baked pie with some extra ghee or olive oil if you like. Use the chile only if you enjoy the extra pungency.

FOR FIERY DIGESTION: Omit the asafoetida and chile. Choose the Vegetable Pie cooking method over the pan-fried pancakes to minimize the chances of acidic digestion.

1. Wash the soaked yellow split mung dal until the water runs clear; drain well. Place them in a food processor along with the water and blend for 2 minutes, or until smooth. Add the ginger, chile, lime juice, masala, salt, turmeric, and asafoetida, if using. Pulse to mix well. Transfer the batter to a large bowl.

2. Fold in the carrots, zucchini, red cabbage, spinach, cilantro, and mint. The batter should be medium-thick, without any excess water

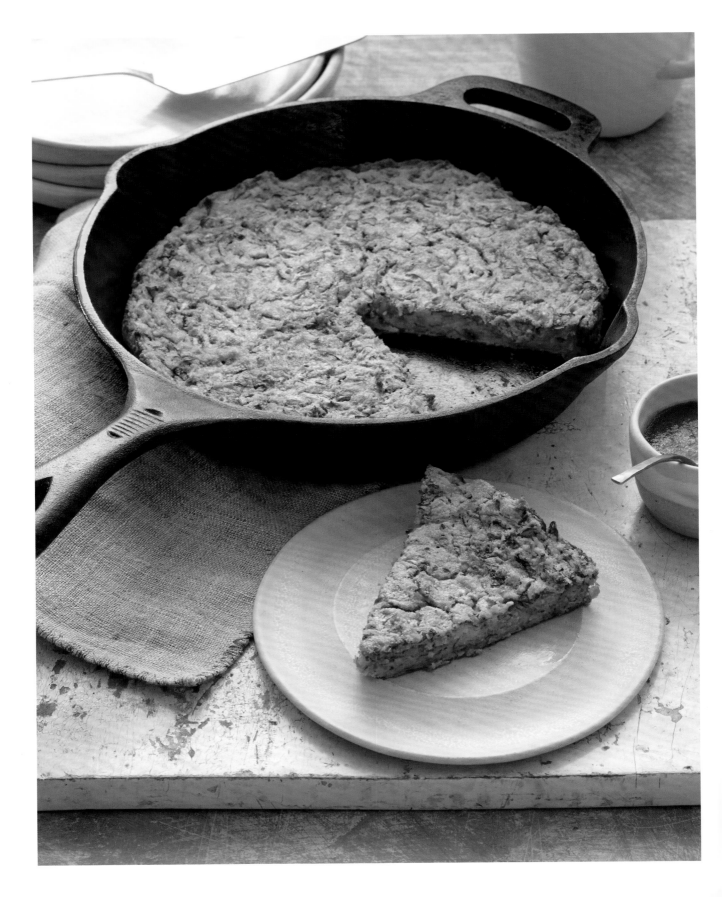

on the sides. If the batter is too thick, add a little more water; if it is too runny, add a little more grated carrot.

RUSTIC VEGETABLE PIE

1. Preheat the oven to 350°F.

2. Heat a well-seasoned 10-inch cast-iron skillet over medium-high heat to medium hot. Generously brush the pan surface with ghee and pour in the batter—it should be about 2 inches deep. Cook the pie uncovered for about 5 minutes, until the edges of the pie become slightly crusty and begin to separate from the pan.

3. Transfer the pie, still in the skillet, to the oven and bake for 10 minutes, then brush the pie surface with ghee, increase the heat to 400°F, and continue to bake for another 10 minutes, or until the top forms an attractive golden crust.

4. Remove from the oven and let the pie cool down and firm up for 10 to 15 minutes, then cut into 8 pieces. Transfer the pie slices to a cooling rack or a serving plate.

CREPE-LIKE PANCAKES

1. Heat a 10-inch (or larger) cast-iron griddle over medium-high heat, brush the surface of the pan with a thin layer of ghee, and, using a ladle, immediately pour a scant ¼ cup batter into the skillet; using the bottom of the ladle, quickly spread the batter into a circle that is as thin as possible (about 3 millimeters). Cook until the bottom is golden and the edges begin to lift from the pan, 3 to 4 minutes. Sprinkle a few drops of ghee on the pancake, then flip it and cook until the second side is golden and firmer, another 2 to 3 minutes. Don't worry if the second side looks more unevenly cooked than the first side—that's just the character of this pancake: smoother at first but turning rough later. Brush a few drops of ghee around the edges of the pancake to make it easier to gently scrape it from the pan. When both sides are cooked, fold the pancake in half, with the first cooked side on the outside.

2. Repeat with remaining batter, adding more ghee as needed. If the pan gets too hot and the ghee starts smoking or if the pancakes are done on the outside but raw on the inside, reduce the heat to low.

3. Serve the pancakes hot with a chutney or sauce or as a side to vegetables and salad.

NOTES

- If you don't have a cast-iron pan to bake the pie, use a Pyrex or similar oven-safe baking dish lined with parchment paper; skip the stovetop cooking and put it straight into the oven.

- If you're not going to eat the pancakes right away, you can spread them on a baking sheet and keep them warm in a preheated 200°F oven until you're ready to serve.

- When cooking pancakes, I find a ½-inch cast-iron griddle and a sharp-edged stainless steel spatula to be the best tools for flipping. Use a deep cast-iron skillet for the pie version.

IRRESISTIBLE BUCKWHEAT CAKE

PREP: 10 MINUTES ▪ **BAKE:** 20 MINUTES   makes 6 to 8 pieces `GF` `DF`

This is an adapted version of a recipe that my friend Dita Simo gave me years ago. When I first tasted this cake, I could not believe that it was gluten-free and dairy-free, and without a drop of cocoa, as it looks like chocolate cake! I like the crunchy contrast of the slivered almonds topping this spongy cake.

I included Irresistible Buckwheat Cake in this chapter because it is perhaps one of the most balancing cakes for when you're feeling Earthy; nevertheless, please exercise self-control and do not indulge in more than one piece at a time. Serve it with Ginger Mint Limeade (page 89), Earthy Digestive Tea (page 87), or Sugar-Down Tea (page 87) for handling the sweetness with ease.

1 cup buckwheat flour

½ cup Sucanat

2 tablespoons arrowroot powder

¾ teaspoon ground cinnamon

¾ teaspoon baking powder

¼ teaspoon baking soda

½ cup coconut oil

½ cup finely chopped dates

⅓ cup raw applesauce (see Note)

½ cup almond milk (page 216)

¼ cup slivered almonds, for decoration

FOR AIRY AND FIERY DIGESTION: Enjoy as is occasionally.

1. Preheat the oven to 375°F. Grease a 9-inch round or square cake pan with coconut oil.

2. In a large bowl, mix together the buckwheat flour, Sucanat, arrowroot powder, ground cinnamon, baking powder, and baking soda.

3. In a food processor, combine the coconut oil, dates, and applesauce and process to a puree, then add the almond milk and pulse to mix.

4. Add the liquid mixture to the dry mixture and stir to create a moist, smooth batter. Spread the batter into the baking pan and sprinkle the slivered almonds on top. Bake for 20 minutes, or until a toothpick or skewer inserted in the middle of the cake comes out clean.

5. Let the cake cool down in the pan, then cut into six or eight pieces. Store covered at room temperature for up to 24 hours.

NOTE

▪ To make raw applesauce, peel and slice an apple and puree it in a small food processor or blender until smooth.

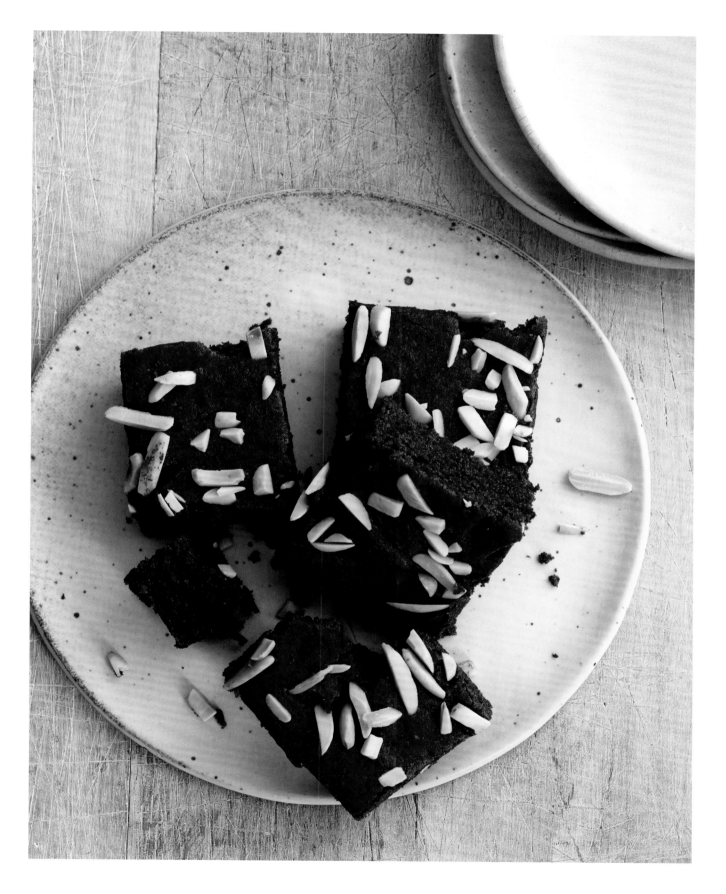

SESAME HONEY BALLS

PREP: 15 MINUTES   makes twelve 1-inch balls `GF` `DF`

How about eating sweets to lose weight? This dessert does just that—when eaten in moderation, of course. I've met many people on weight-reduction diets who become overwhelmed with sugar cravings. Foods of sweet taste usually contribute to building bodily tissues and go against weight loss, but honey is an exception. Raw honey reduces earthy energy and sesame detoxifies fat tissue—you can enjoy them together as a sweet treat without fear.

   These soft and slightly grainy Sesame Honey Balls will bring a variety of tastes to your palate, from sweet to slightly bitter. When including them in a meal, consider that sesame seeds become incompatible for digestion when eaten with meat or milk.

½ cup plus 2 tablespoons hulled (white) sesame seeds, plus more for topping if you like

⅔ cup almond meal or almond pulp (well-squeezed) from making almond milk

¾ teaspoon ground cardamom

½ teaspoon vanilla extract

½ teaspoon lime or orange zest (optional)

¼ cup raw honey (crystalized honey is best)

> **FOR AIRY DIGESTION:** Enjoy as is occasionally.
>
> **FOR FIERY DIGESTION:** These are probably too heating for you (both honey and sesame are quite heating)—so have just a bite.

1. In a small skillet, dry-toast the sesame seeds over medium-low heat to a light tan color, shaking or stirring the pan frequently, about 3 minutes.

2. In a food processor, finely grind the toasted sesame seeds with the almond pulp, cardamom, vanilla, and zest, if using. Transfer to a medium bowl, add the honey, and mix well with a spoon to a sticky consistency that will hold when shaped into a ball.

3. Roll the mixture into 1-inch balls. You can decorate them with a dimple of toasted sesame seeds if you like.

4. To store, keep refrigerated in a closed container for up to 4 days.

VARIATION

■ Replace the almond pulp with ⅔ cup sunflower seeds, soaked for 1 hour and well drained.

The Healing Benefits of Sesame

Sesame is of bitter, sweet, and astringent tastes and of heating, oily, and heavy qualities. When combined with daily exercise, sesame seeds can help the body eliminate fat-soluble toxins through the sweat glands. Sesame is rich in calcium, iron, and antioxidants. It is excellent for strengthening our bones, teeth, and hair. Do not eat more than 3 tablespoons sesame seeds a day.

EARTHY DIGESTIVE TEA

COOK: 5 MINUTES   serves 1 GF DF

This is a quick but effective remedy for slow (Earthy) digestion or after overeating. When you feel that your stomach is acting lazy and your meal is still sitting in there, this tea will come to the rescue. Sip it warm after lunch and dinner.

1 teaspoon grated fresh ginger

1½ teaspoons chopped fresh mint leaves, or ½ teaspoon dried mint

Bring 1 cup water to a boil in a small saucepan over medium-high heat. Add the ginger and mint, reduce the heat, cover, and simmer for 10 minutes. Strain and sip slowly.

SUGAR-DOWN TEA BLEND

COOK: 10 MINUTES   makes about 2 tablespoons, enough for 5 cups of tea GF DF

This bitter-pungent tea reduces sugar cravings and supports the body in converting carbohydrates into energy. Sip it after eating foods of sweet taste and when you need to lower your blood sugar. (If you are on blood sugar medication, please consult with your doctor before drinking this tea.) When taken thirty minutes before a meal, this tea increases appetite. Look for gymnema leaf in stores that sell loose herbs or online.

1 teaspoon gymnema leaf

1 teaspoon dried rose petals or 1 dried rose bud

1 teaspoon coriander seeds

2 cardamom pods

2 whole cloves

½ teaspoon cinnamon granules or crushed cinnamon stick

½ teaspoon powdered ginger

¼ teaspoon ground nutmeg

¼ teaspoon fenugreek seeds

Pulse all the ingredients in a spice grinder to crush them. Store in an airtight container, away from light.

To make a serving of tea: Bring 1 cup water to a boil in a small saucepan over medium-high heat. Add the tea blend, reduce the heat, cover, and simmer for 3 minutes. Strain and sip slowly.

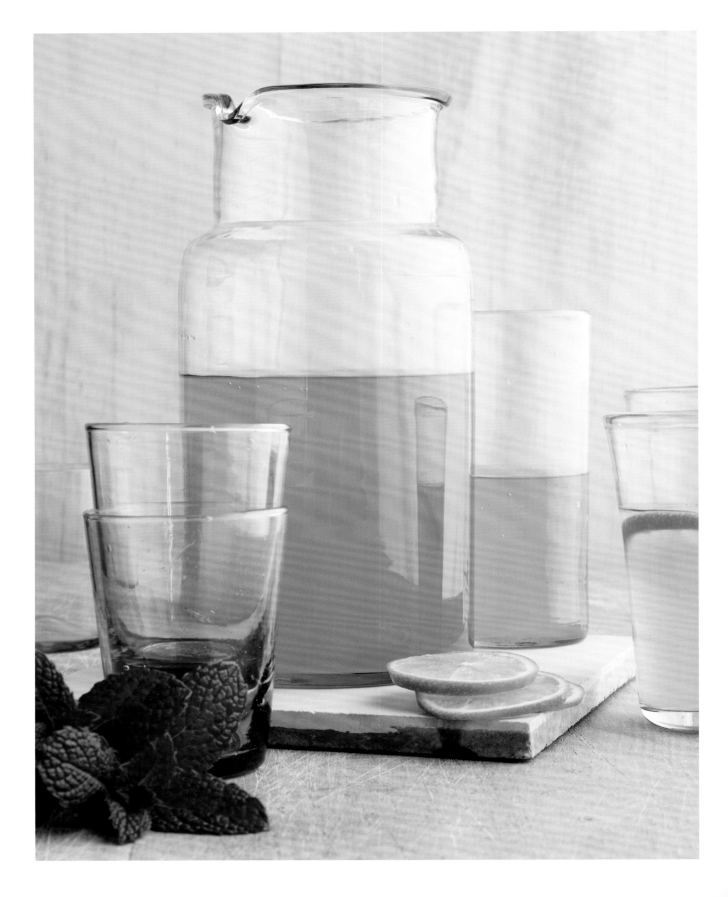

GINGER MINT LIMEADE

PREP: 10 TO 12 MINUTES

makes a little more than 1 quart GF DF

We've been serving this drink for years at Bhagavat Life events, enjoying the usual remark: "You should bottle this stuff and sell it."

Sharp ginger makes your taste buds tingle; that's why you need to tame it a smidge with lime, mint, and sugar. Ginger Mint Limeade will help you digest any meal, but I like to serve it in cool weather.

4 cups spring or filtered water

3 tablespoons minced fresh ginger (no need to peel)

¼ cup plus 1 tablespoon fresh lime juice (2 or 3 limes)

1 cup loosely packed chopped fresh mint (with stems)

¼ cup plus 1 tablespoon raw sugar (one that is light in color)

FOR AIRY DIGESTION: Drink as is or add a little more water to reduce its pungency.

FOR FIERY DIGESTION: This beverage might be too heating for you. In your balanced Fiery state, you may enjoy this drink diluted with 1 cup extra water.

1. In a blender, blend 2 cups of the water with the remaining ingredients.

2. Strain through a cheesecloth or nut milk bag—squeeze out as much juice as you can.

3. Add the remaining 2 cups water, stir, and serve.

The Healing Benefits of Ginger

Ayurveda calls ginger the "universal medicine"—it is good for so many ailments! Ginger is pungent, heating, and invigorating for digestion and circulation, but not as stimulating as other hot condiments such as chiles, onions, or garlic. Modern studies have confirmed that ginger supports immunity, reduces inflammation, and maintains good digestion.

Ginger is available in three common forms: fresh, dry (as root or powder), and sunthi (Ayurvedic cured dried ginger). Fresh ginger is quite heating, and it is most balancing when you're feeling Airy or Earthy. Ginger powder is best when you're feeling very Earthy because of its heating and drying properties.

Nowadays regular dry ginger is often mistaken for sunthi, but the classical Ayurvedic texts draw a clear distinction between the two: regular dry ginger is simply the dehydrated version of the fresh root; sunthi, on the other hand, has been cured before dehydration and is a lot less drying and heating. When mixed properly with other spices, sunthi is the best form of ginger for when you're feeling Fiery and in the summer. It is also very effective in increasing breast milk for nursing mothers. Sunthi is available at www.chandika.com.

SUGGESTED ENERGIZING MENUS

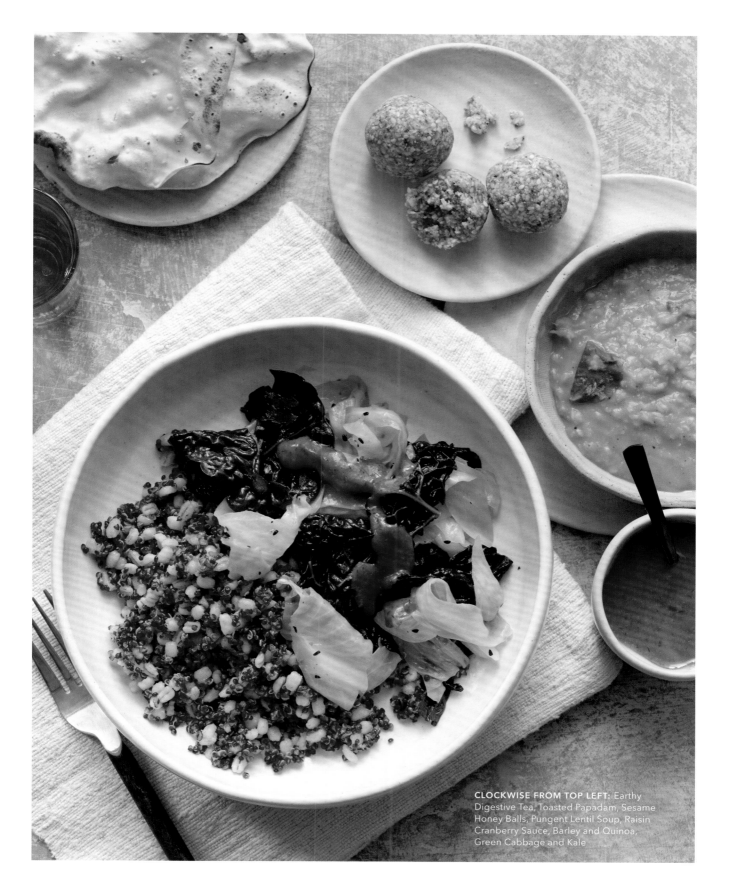

CLOCKWISE FROM TOP LEFT: Earthy Digestive Tea, Toasted Papadam, Sesame Honey Balls, Pungent Lentil Soup, Raisin Cranberry Sauce, Barley and Quinoa, Green Cabbage and Kale

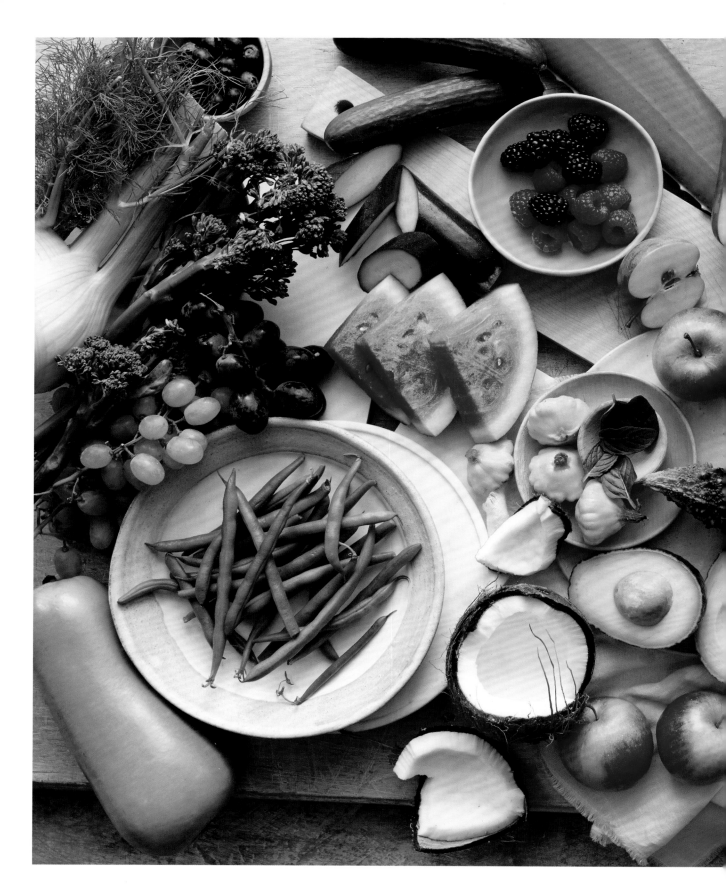

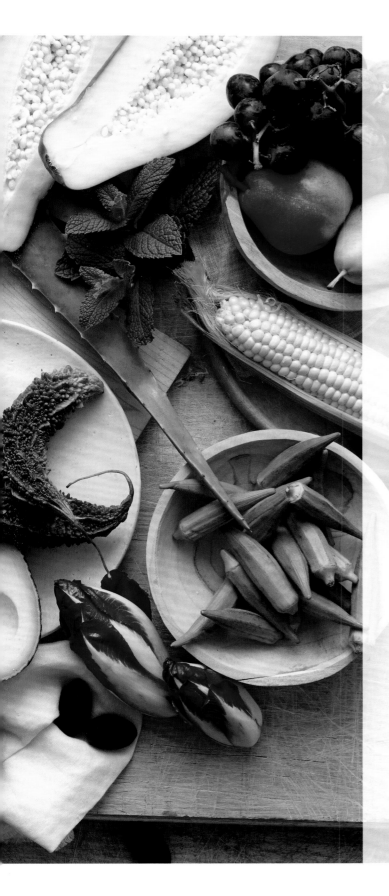

SUMMER
&
EARLY FALL

COOLING RECIPES

In summer, temperatures can rise up to 105'F and more in many places even in temperate regions. This is the time to lighten up on clothing and enjoy lots of outdoor activities, travel, and vacation. Whatever we do, work or play, we all experience the effects of hot weather: burning and sweaty skin, dehydration, and midday fatigue.

If you are a Fiery person, summer is probably the toughest season for you. At times you may feel as if your blood is boiling! Have you noticed a special reflux or skin rash that appears only in summer? If you do, it's probably a reaction from not balancing your Fiery digestion with cooling foods.

Some of us may experience irregular Airy digestion in summer—the body feels really hot but digestive fire is low; you are not so hungry, but when you do eat you are not satisfied with food. This is where it gets tricky, because foods and spices that generally enhance digestive fire such as ginger, chiles, and cinnamon are also very heating and will perpetuate Fiery aggravation. In this case, SV Ayurveda recommends avoiding the heating spices and instead moderately seasoning summer dishes with fennel, coriander, cloves, a little turmeric, and fresh herbs.

Balance with vibrant cooked and raw foods of the summer harvest: cooling (summer squash, fennel, all greens, coconut, cucumber, lime, mint), liquid and hydrating (coconut water, aloe vera juice), and the light, calming qualities of sweet, bitter, and astringent tastes (see "The Six Tastes of Food" on page 249) to control your heightened metabolism. In this way your body will dry up excessive moisture accumulated in spring, and the carbs from fruits and vegetables will support your high-energy activities in summer.

Coconut in all its variations is a wonderful food to enjoy in this season. If you have sharp Fiery digestion, organic virgin coconut oil is your best cooking oil. You can also drizzle it on hot food, but do not eat it straight out of the jar or with raw foods, because cold coconut oil is more likely to cause blockages. If you have irregular or slow digestion in summer, then the best way for you to receive the medicinal cooling benefits of coconut oil is by massaging it into your skin. In this case, ghee (which has more Fiery energy) would be your best cooking oil option.

In general keep this cooling diet through early fall, until the temperatures start dropping below 65°F, to assist your body with the transformation of accumulated heat during the transition from summer to autumn.

Please note that iced foods and beverages do not fall into the "cooling foods" category. Drinking iced beverages or eating ice cream may give you immediate relief from the scorching heat, but it will gradually shrink and damage your digestive channels. That's why Ayurveda (and almost all holistic medicine traditions) strongly advises us against eating iced foods even in summer.

Stay away from foods that are heating as well as high sulfur foods (chiles, ginger, hot sauce, tomatoes, onions, garlic, asafoetida, black salt); heavy (proteins, wheat) and dry foods (crackers, yeasted bread, large beans); deep-fried foods, coffee, and alcohol; and acidic foods (sour cream, store-bought yogurt, vinegar, lemon, soy sauce, pickles, fermented cheese, egg yolks); reduce foods of sour, salty, and pungent tastes (see "The Six Tastes of Food" on page 249).

Avoid detoxing in this season unless recommended by an expert and under close supervision. Cleansing in summer may overheat your liver and lead to unpleasant healing crises.

TIPS FOR IMPROVING FIERY DIGESTION

Please revisit "Setting the Stage for Your Meals: It's Not Just What You Eat, But How You Eat It" on pages 40-41—this practice is always useful, no matter what your digestion is and how it's behaving. Because millions of people today suffer from hyperacidity, the guidelines below target overcoming acid reflux and heartburn (common reactions in sharp Fiery digestion). I've seen many of my students and clients improve by following these tips to the point that their doctor was able to take them off antacid medication. (If you experience irregular Airy digestion in summer, read the tips on page 141.)

- Follow the recipes and recommendations in this chapter.

- Chew ½ teaspoon After-Meal Spice Blend for Fiery Digestion (at right) after every meal.

- Eat four to five times a day. Never skip or delay meals (eat appropriate snacks such as sweet, juicy fruit if you get hungry between meals).

- As soon as you wake up, have a Cooked Apple Pre-Breakfast (page 143).

- Eat lunch by 12 p.m.

- Finish eating dinner by 6 p.m.—this recommendation has been proven helpful by numerous gastrointestinal doctors.

- Make sure to have enough protein for dinner, as it is highly balancing for Fiery types to consume a good-quality, easy-to-digest protein dish at night. Try my Creamy Green Protein Soup (page 107) or Stuffed Avocados with Fresh Cheese (page 122).

- If you get hungry after dinner, drink at least ½ cup Fennel Milk (page 135) before bedtime.

- Drink room-temperature water throughout the day.

- Drink fresh coconut water.

- Never drink coffee or alcohol on an empty stomach (best to avoid them completely as they are acidic and heating)

- Favor Soma Salt (see page 46), the most cooling of all salts, and reduce salt in general in your food.

- Go for a walk early in the morning and at night—at sunrise and moonrise (the moon rays are very cooling and calming); avoid direct exposure to sun between 10 a.m. and 2 p.m.

- Go to bed by 10 p.m.

AFTER-MEAL SPICE BLEND FOR FIERY DIGESTION

Although fennel enhances digestive fire, its sweet, licorice-like taste balances the pungency of the spice so that it does not overheat the body. Toasting the fennel also reduces its slightly heating properties, thus making it an especially helpful spice for when you're feeling Fiery. In large quantities, however, fennel can be heating, so do not overdo it.

This home remedy may help you alleviate symptoms of indigestion, but it cannot replace poor diet. Good food is the foundation for good digestion.

4 tablespoons fennel seeds

In a small heavy skillet, dry-toast the fennel seeds over low heat until they darken a few shades and release their aroma; remove from the pan and let them cool down completely. Store in an airtight jar for up to a month. Chew ½ teaspoon after every meal.

BARLEY FLAKES BREAKFAST

PREP: 10 MINUTES ▪ **COOK:** 5 MINUTES   serves 2 `GF` `DF`

I am a big fan of whole-grain flakes for breakfast—they are grounding yet light and filling enough to keep you going till lunch. Flakes are basically pressed whole grains. Pressing keeps their nutritious bran intact but makes them quick to cook and easy to digest. Prentiss, my charming husband of Fiery persuasion, prefers savory tastes for breakfast, and Barley Flakes Breakfast is one dish he enjoys. I like adding nori because it is rich in minerals and lends a layer of flavor, color, and chewiness to this otherwise plain dish.

   If you only have fifteen minutes to cook lunch, go ahead and make barley flakes as your grain dish and serve them with salad, leafy greens, or vegetables. Barley flakes are sold in health food stores and online.

2 teaspoons ghee, coconut oil, or olive oil

2 green cardamom pods, slightly opened on one side

⅛ teaspoon ground turmeric

2 curry leaves (optional)

¼ teaspoon ground cumin

1 cup barley flakes

1½ cups water

¾ teaspoon salt

½ sheet toasted nori (8½ x 7½ inches), torn into 1-inch pieces

Splash of lime juice

FOR AIRY DIGESTION: Add 1 teaspoon olive oil after you remove the flakes from the heat; add an additional ¼ cup water while cooking if you'd like the dish creamier.

FOR EARTHY DIGESTION: Reduce the oil to 1 teaspoon; add ¼ teaspoon freshly ground black pepper before you add the nori. For variety, replace barley flakes with rye flakes.

1. In a 1- to 2-quart saucepan, heat the ghee over low heat. Add the cardamom pods, turmeric, and curry leaves, if using, and cook for 3 to 4 seconds, until they release their aroma. Add the cumin, followed immediately by the barley flakes. Stir well to allow the flakes to absorb the oil and spices.

2. Add the water and salt, increase the heat, and bring to a boil. Reduce the heat to low, cover, and simmer for about 5 minutes, until the flakes have absorbed all the water and look soft and fluffy.

3. Turn off the heat, remove the cardamom pods, and add the nori; mix and fluff the flakes with a fork. Sprinkle with a little lime juice to enhance digestion and taste. Add 1 or 2 tablespoons water if you find the flakes too thick. Serve hot.

- **Add-ons:** For a more sumptuous meal, serve Barley Flakes Breakfast with slices of avocado (for the Airy), sliced raw red radish or celery sticks (for the Fiery), or a spicy pickle or sauce (for the Earthy)—these are just a few ideas. Play with this recipe and see what else you'd like to add. Just remember not to combine this savory barley recipe with milk because milk and salt are incompatible for digestion.

- **Gluten-free option:** Substitute flat rice (sold in Indian grocery stores) or gluten-free rolled oats for the barley flakes.

The Healing Benefits of Barley

Barley is an ancient grain that has been prepared by cooks throughout the world for thousands of years. Barley flakes or hulled (not pearled) barley are most nutritious. Ayurveda includes barley in remedies for numerous conditions including weight loss, water retention, weakness, recovery from prolonged illness, ulcers, dull complexion, sore throat, cough, and loss of voice. With its cooling, sweet, rough, and slightly astringent qualities, barley is an excellent balancing grain for when you're feeling Earthy or Fiery. Here are more of barley's benefits:

- It is as an effective "fertilizer" for friendly bacteria in the gut.

- It acts as a binder of toxins in the colon and blood.

- It regulates blood sugar for up to ten hours after eating.

- It lowers cholesterol.

- It is abundant in fiber, thus supporting timely formation and elimination of wastes.

- It heals chronic diarrhea with mucus.

- It calms down an inflamed urinary tract.

- Barley has a bit of gluten, but much less than wheat. Many people who react to wheat have no digestive problems with organic barley. Of course, if you have celiac disease, you have to avoid barley completely.

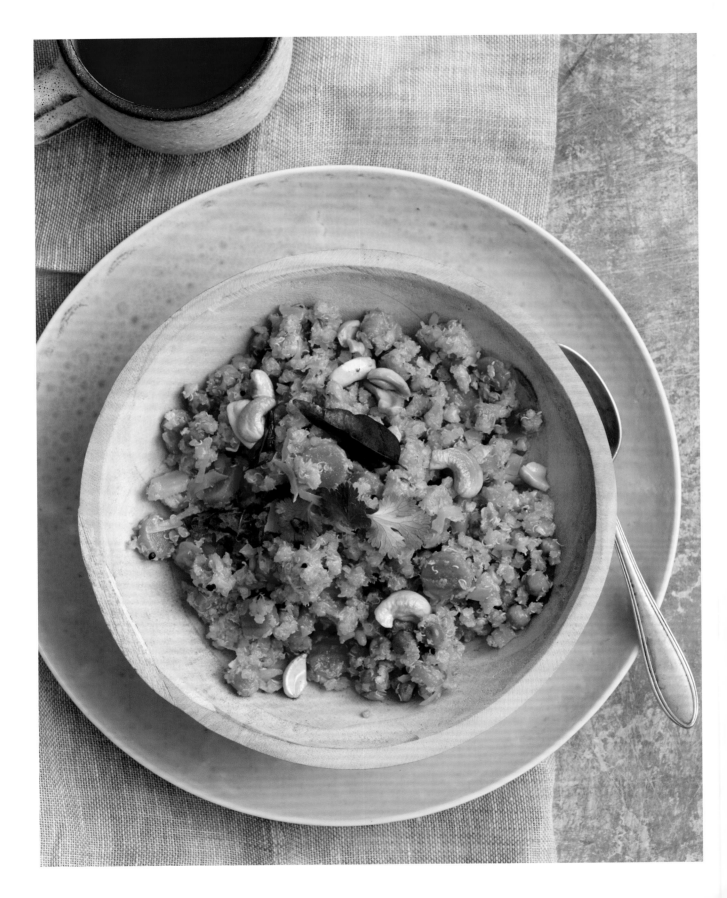

QUINOA FLAKES AND VEGETABLE UPMA

PREP: 5 MINUTES ▪ **COOK:** 20 MINUTES   serves 2 `GF` `DF`

Upma (aka uppittu) is a traditional Indian dish of semolina and vegetables fried with spices; it resembles a fluffy-textured Italian polenta. Regarded with great affection in yoga circles and Ayurvedic schools, upma is a satisfying meal, quick to fix for yourself and easy to prepare in large quantities.

I meet many people who are sensitive to wheat and gluten; this gluten-free take on upma substitutes nutritious and fast-cooking quinoa flakes for the semolina. It is a little stickier in consistency but still tasty and flavorful. This dish is great for using up fresh vegetables that you have on hand. I really like the sulfury nuance of cabbage—that's why I list it as a main ingredient—but you can make this upma with just about any vegetable.

Quinoa Flakes and Vegetable Upma makes a filling breakfast, but with a tossed green salad and chutney, you have a complete lunch or dinner to share with a guest or family. Raisin-Cranberry Sauce (page 189) or Cilantro Chutney (page 191) go especially well with this dish.

2 tablespoons ghee or coconut oil

1 cup quinoa flakes

¼ teaspoon ground turmeric

¼ teaspoon cumin seeds

¼ teaspoon kalonji seeds

1 teaspoon yellow split mung dal (optional)

6 curry leaves

½ teaspoon powdered sunthi ginger
(see page 89) or 1 teaspoon grated
fresh ginger

¾ teaspoon salt

1 cup grated green cabbage or kohlrabi

½ cup finely chopped vegetables such as
carrot, zucchini, fennel, daikon radish,
green beans, broccoli, and/or cauliflower

⅓ cup fresh or frozen petite peas

GARNISHES

2 tablespoons slivered almonds, pistachios,
or cashew pieces

1 teaspoon ghee or coconut oil

¼ teaspoon Cooling Pungent Masala
(page 222), or to taste

2 tablespoons fresh cilantro leaves

1 tablespoon fresh lime juice

FOR AIRY DIGESTION: Choose more grounding vegetables such as carrots, daikon radish, taro root, and zucchini.

FOR EARTHY DIGESTION: Reduce the ghee to 2 teaspoons in Steps 1 and 2. Add 1 or 2 seeded and minced green Thai chiles along with the ginger in Step 2. In Step 5, omit the nuts and substitute Fat-Burning Masala (page 218) for the Cooling Pungent Masala.

1. Heat 1 tablespoon of the ghee in a heavy 2-quart sauté pan over medium-low heat. Add the quinoa flakes and toast for 2 to 3 minutes, until the flakes absorb the oil, darken a shade, and become slightly crisp. Transfer to a small bowl and set aside.

2. Wipe the pan and heat the remaining 1 tablespoon ghee over low heat. Add the turmeric and toast until it darkens a shade and releases its aroma, about 15 seconds. Add the cumin, kalonji, and mung dal and continue to cook for another 5 to 10 seconds for the seeds and lentils to release their flavor. Add the curry leaves and ginger, cook for

5 to 10 seconds, then add the salt, cabbage, other vegetables, and peas. Increase the heat to medium and stir-fry the vegetables until they are well coated in the seasonings and become a bit limp, 2 to 3 minutes (if the mixture is too dry, add 1 tablespoon water to prevent burning). Reduce the heat to low, cover, and continue to cook, stirring occasionally, until the vegetables are crisp-tender, 3 to 4 minutes.

3. While the vegetables are cooking, toast the nuts in a small pan with 1 teaspoon ghee over low heat until they turn golden, about 2 minutes. Set aside.

4. Carefully pour 2 cups boiling hot water over the vegetables. Slowly stir in the toasted quinoa flakes. Increase the heat to medium-low and cook, stirring often, until all of the liquid is absorbed and the upma is of a sticky yet somewhat fluffy texture, 1 to 2 minutes. Turn off the heat and cover for about 5 minutes.

5. Garnish with the toasted nuts, masala, cilantro leaves, and a sprinkle of lime juice just before serving.

VARIATION

- Add 2 tablespoons dried shredded coconut when you add the quinoa flakes in Step 1.

BASMATI RICE AND RED QUINOA

SOAK: 30 MINUTES ▪ **COOK:** 20 MINUTES

serves 4 GF DF

Perhaps you've never thought of cooking these two grains together, but they are the perfect match. The tall and soft basmati grains dance with the round and rough quinoa seeds, surrounded by the aroma of dill—it's a date! This grain dish goes well with vegetables, salads, and chutneys.

½ cup red quinoa, soaked for 30 minutes in water to cover

½ cup white basmati rice

1 teaspoon salt

3 teaspoons ghee or coconut oil

1 to 2 tablespoons pine nuts or chopped walnuts (optional)

2 tablespoons minced fresh dill

FOR AIRY DIGESTION: Add another teaspoon or two of ghee in Step 3.

FOR EARTHY DIGESTION: Omit the ghee in Step 3.

1. Using a mesh strainer, rinse the soaked quinoa and rice until the water runs clear. Set aside to drain.

2. In a 1- to 2-quart saucepan, bring 2 cups water to a boil and add the salt.

3. Add the rice, quinoa, and 1 teaspoon of the ghee and return to a boil. Cover with a tight-fitting lid, reduce the heat to low, and gently simmer for 15 to 20 minutes. Do not open or stir the pot. In 15 minutes, check if the grains need a little more water or more time: a grain of rice should not be hard when squeezed between your two fingers, and for the quinoa you should see a little white sprout (like a tail) separating from the seed.

4. Turn off the heat. Add the remaining ghee and the pine nuts, if using. Cover and let the grains firm up for 5 more minutes.

5. Sprinkle the minced dill to garnish and fluff with a fork. Serve steamy hot.

NOTES

▪ Adding ghee or oil to the grains as they cook helps them remain separate and light.

▪ Cooking rice with ghee or oil is important because fat helps digest the starch in grains.

VARIATION

▪ Substitute white, black, or tricolor quinoa for the red quinoa.

COOLING BASMATI RICE

SOAK: 30 MINUTES ▪ **COOK:** ABOUT 15 MINUTES

serves 4 to 5 **GF** **DF**

This recipe offers the best way to enjoy white rice for those concerned about blood sugar. The ingredients are really simple, but this method of washing, soaking, and cooking the white basmati rice lowers its glycemic index and helps keep blood sugar levels down. Blood sugar commonly spikes from consuming processed sugars in foods or drinks such as cereals or sodas or eating too many starchy foods that get digested too quickly. Eating Cooling Basmati Rice prepared this way slows down the digestion of the starch, so spikes should be minimal if any. It is important to choose the basmati variety for this dish, as any other type of white rice will not have the same healing effect.

1 cup white basmati rice

1 teaspoon salt

1 teaspoon ghee or coconut oil

3 to 4 tablespoons chopped fresh dill, cilantro, or parsley

FOR AIRY DIGESTION: Increase the ghee or coconut oil to 1 tablespoon in Step 4.

FOR EARTHY DIGESTION: Add 4 slightly crushed cardamom pods and 4 peppercorns in Step 2.

1. To wash and soak the rice: Place the rice in a strainer and dip it in a bowl of cold water. Wash the grains by gently rubbing them between your fingertips. Do not crush the grains! Lift the strainer, empty and refill the bowl with water, and repeat 2 or 3 times, until the washing water runs more or less clear. Keeping the rice in the strainer, soak it in a bowl of water for 30 minutes, then drain.

2. Bring 6 cups water to a boil; add the salt and rice. Cook uncovered over medium heat for 10 to 15 minutes. Check if the rice is ready by pressing a grain between your fingers—the grain should be whole and soft without any grainy feeling.

3. Turn off the heat. Immediately pour the cooked rice through a strainer or colander to drain away all the water (this will take away additional starch that otherwise would quickly convert into sugar).

4. Pour the drained rice back into the pot, quickly drizzle in the ghee, and leave the pot covered for at least 5 minutes to allow the hot grains to firm up.

5. Garnish with the fresh dill and fluff it up with a big fork. Serve steamy hot.

NOTE

▪ The biggest failure you can have with this recipe is overcooking the rice into a big mushy flop. To avoid that, use a timer in Steps 1 and 2.

COOLING KHICHARI

SOAK: 30 MINUTES ▪ **PREP:** 5 MINUTES ▪ **COOK:** ABOUT 30 MINUTES   serves 4 GF DF

This creamy, porridge-like blend has been a centerpiece in Ayurvedic cuisine for centuries—it has been used to nourish the sick and the healthy, babies and the elderly, for regular meals or during special periods of detox. Khichari is simple yet very soothing and nourishing and can be eaten for breakfast, lunch, or dinner. Honestly, this dish is my meal savior when I have only half an hour to cook.

Many of my students have told me amazing khichari stories—how this dish helped them eat well through a period of financial crisis (yes, khichari is most inexpensive!); how it saved one from colon surgery (the last medical resort for ulcerative colitis); how it cleared a deviated septum; or how it helped a novice cook build her confidence in the kitchen. There is some hidden magic behind the simplicity of this "pot of gold." I hope you will fall in love with the khichari recipes in my book and become the khichari expert in your neighborhood!

1 cup yellow split mung dal

1 cup basmati rice or quinoa

6 cups hot water

1 cup diced vegetables, such as daikon radish, carrots, asparagus, taro root, zucchini, broccoli, cauliflower, and/or kale (optional)

1 tablespoon ghee or olive oil

6 fresh curry leaves or 2 cassia leaves

1 teaspoon ground fennel seeds

½ teaspoon powdered sunthi ginger (see page 89) or 1 teaspoon grated fresh ginger

½ teaspoon ground turmeric

2 teaspoons salt

1 tablespoon olive oil

GARNISHES

¼ cup chopped fresh cilantro, basil, dill, or parsley

4 lime wedges

FOR AIRY DIGESTION: Add freshly ground black pepper along with the salt in Step 3.

FOR EARTHY DIGESTION: Substitute quinoa for the rice; add 1 or 2 seeded and minced green Thai chiles along with the vegetables in Step 2.

1. Soak the mung dal for 30 minutes, then drain, wash well, and drain again. Wash and drain the basmati rice.

2. Combine the mung dal, rice, and water in a heavy 4-quart saucepan. Bring to a full boil over high heat, stirring occasionally and removing any froth from the surface. Add the vegetables, ghee, curry leaves, fennel, ginger, and turmeric and mix well. (Add quick-cooking vegetables such as zucchini, asparagus, or leafy greens 15 minutes into boiling the khichari.) Reduce the heat to medium-low, cover with a tight-fitting lid, and simmer gently for 20 minutes, or until the mung dal and rice are soft and fully cooked, stirring occasionally to prevent them from

sticking to the bottom of the pot. If the khichari starts to dry out, add more water.

3. Turn off the heat and add the salt and olive oil. Serve garnished with the fresh herbs and lime wedges.

NOTES

- For more protein, substitute 1 cup chana dal, aka split chickpeas (soaked for at least 4 hours or overnight) for the mung dal. Cook the chana on its own in 6 cups water for 20 minutes, or until it is soft and begins to break apart. Then add the rest of the ingredients in Step 2. Chana dal is available in Indian grocery stores.

- If you eat this khichari as a part of a cleanse, add more water to bring it to a soupy consistency; reduce the salt by half or omit it altogether. Less or no salt supports elimination.

- If you're not cleansing, feel free to substitute red lentils for the yellow split mung dal or use a combination of the two.

The Healing and Detox Benefits of Khichari

- It's a complete protein. There is no coincidence that the combination of rice and beans has been a staple around the world for thousands of years. Grains and legumes contain partial amino acids on their own. When eaten together (as in khichari), rice and beans provide all the essential amino acids for nutritionally sustainable meals, perfect for those on a plant-based diet.

- It helps burn body fat while keeping blood sugar stable. Many water fasts or juice cleanses strain and deplete blood sugar reserves, which can make you extremely hungry or irritable and give you severe headaches. While one of the goals of a fast is to shift the body into fat-burning metabolism, this will not happen if the body is under stress and strain as a result of an extreme fast. On a khichari cleanse day, you are eating a delicious complete protein dish three times a day, so there is no starvation response whatsoever. Dr. John Douillard, a renowned Ayurvedic practitioner and author, advises us that if we are straining or hungry during a cleanse, we are not getting the optimal benefits. The more comfortable we are, the more fat we will burn (if we need to burn fat, that is).

- It's nourishing yet easy to digest. White basmati rice, quinoa, and yellow split mung dal are easy to assimilate, placing less of a burden on digestion. It is especially important to use them rather than the other bean options during a cleanse because the metabolism slows down and the digestive strength weakens when cleansing. Heavier brown rice, chana dal, red lentils, or mung beans with the husks may irritate the intestinal wall and cause digestive gas or abdominal pain.

- It helps heal the gut. As it is so easy to digest, khichari heals and soothes the intestinal wall. Stress can often irritate the gut and compromise digestion, which will then make the body more clogged with toxins from indigestion. Eating just khichari allows much of the digestion to be at rest while providing the nutrition needed to heal the gut and nourish the body.

BLACK LENTIL SOUP

SOAK: AT LEAST 1 HOUR ▪ **COOK:** ABOUT 45 MINUTES

serves 4 `GF` `DF`

I really like black (aka beluga) lentils because they are flavorful, easy to digest, and a good source of protein, fiber, and iron. Back when I discovered them some time ago, they were a specialty food, but now they are a common health food store item and can easily be found online. Black lentils have a chewy yet soft texture and hold their shape when cooked; that's why I use them as a substitute for black beans in soups and pâtés.

Black Lentil Soup goes well with Cooling Basmati Rice (page 102) or Basmati Rice and Red Quinoa (page 101), Broccoli with Fresh Cheese (page 115), and any salad.

1 tablespoon ghee or olive oil

1 teaspoon Cooling Pungent Masala (page 222)

1 celery stick, sliced (about ½ cup)

1 cup black lentils, soaked for at least 1 hour or overnight, drained, and rinsed

1½ teaspoons ground coriander

½ teaspoon ground cumin

½ teaspoon dried thyme or savory

1½ teaspoons salt

GARNISHES

1 tablespoon olive oil

2 tablespoons chopped fresh dill or parsley

1 tablespoon fresh lime juice

FOR AIRY DIGESTION: Eat as is.

FOR EARTHY DIGESTION: Add 1 or 2 minced green Thai chiles when you add the celery in Step 1.

1. In a 2-quart saucepan, heat the ghee over medium-low heat and add the masala and celery. Cover, reduce the heat to low, and cook, stirring occasionally to soften the celery without coloring it, about 5 minutes.

2. Add 4 cups water, the lentils, coriander, cumin, thyme, and salt, increase the heat to medium-high, and bring to a boil. Reduce the heat to low, cover, and simmer for about 40 minutes, until the lentils are butter-soft.

3. Remove from the heat. You may partially blend the soup to give it a creamy base; add more water if you like. Spoon into bowls and garnish with the olive oil, dill, and lime juice. Serve hot.

NOTE

▪ A slow cooker will take the flavor and texture of this soup to a whole new level. Use hot water and cook for about 3 hours on high.

VARIATIONS

▪ Substitute fennel or carrots for the celery.

▪ Substitute green, brown, or French lentils for the black lentils.

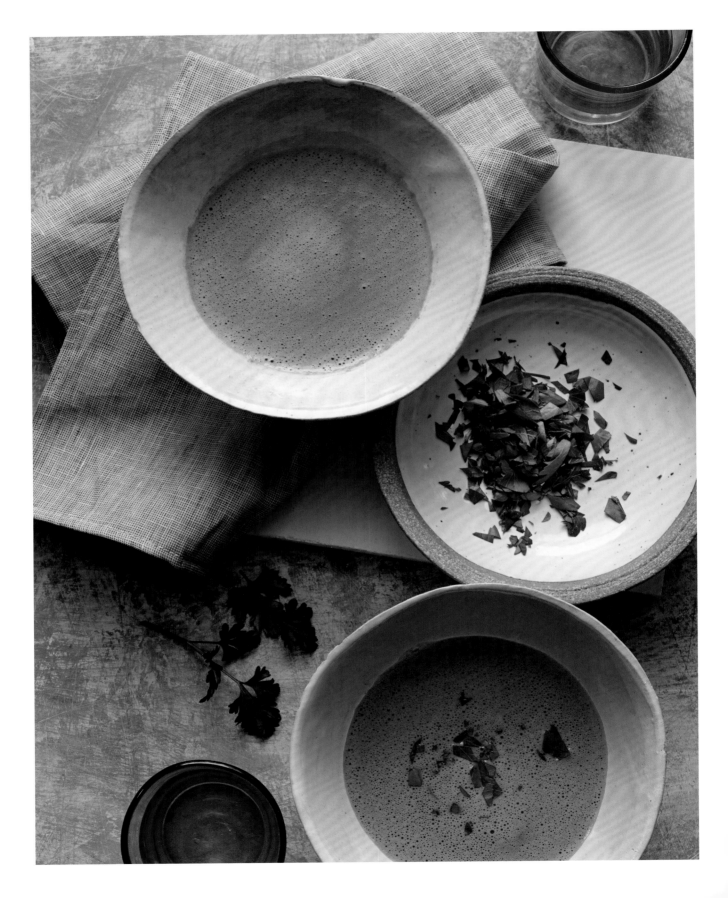

CREAMY GREEN PROTEIN SOUP

PREP: 10 MINUTES (WITH ALREADY MADE CHEESE) ▪ **COOK:** 20 MINUTES   serves 4 `GF` `DF`

I learned this recipe from Vaidya R. K. Mishra, who included it in my autoimmune treatment protocol. It is both nourishing and detoxifying, and when eaten regularly, this quick soup can replenish nutrient deficiencies, boost immunity, and restore vitality. To me, it offered enhanced digestibility of the protein and minerals I was looking for in raw green smoothies.

Creamy Green Protein Soup is suitable for everyone. If you eat it a few times a week, use different greens every time to vary the nutrients and taste.

2 teaspoons ghee or olive oil

1 teaspoon Cooling Masala (page 221)

1 teaspoon salt

¼ teaspoon ground turmeric

⅛ teaspoon fenugreek seeds

1 cup crumbled fresh soft cheese (page 202)

1 pound leafy greens such as chard, beet greens, collards, spinach, kale, and/or amaranth

½ cup fresh parsley leaves

GARNISH

Fresh lime juice

FOR AIRY DIGESTION: Substitute Digestive Masala (page 223) for the Cooling Masala. Add ¼ teaspoon black pepper and a drizzle of olive oil in Step 4.

FOR EARTHY DIGESTION: Substitute Energizing Masala (page 221) for the Cooling Masala. Add 1 tablespoon grated fresh ginger in Step 1.

1. In a 3- to 4-quart saucepan, combine 2 cups water with the ghee, masala, salt, turmeric, fenugreek, and cheese. Bring to a simmer over medium-low heat and cook for 15 minutes.

2. While the cheese is cooking, prep your greens: wash, stem, and tear them—this should yield about 8 packed cups. Gradually add the greens and parsley, turning them over until they wilt but still retain their vibrant green color, 3 to 5 minutes. Turn off the heat and leave the soup uncovered to cool it down a bit.

3. Transfer the soup to a blender and blend to a smooth and creamy consistency. Reheat the soup if needed.

4. Garnish with lime juice and serve hot.

VARIATIONS

▪ **Dairy-free option:** Substitute ½ cup cashews (soaked overnight) or ½ cup rinsed lentils (red, black, or green) or yellow split mung dal for the fresh cheese in Step 1.

▪ Substitute 1 cup of another green vegetable for 2 cups of the greens. Try chopped asparagus, green beans, broccoli, cabbage, zucchini, or lauki squash (see page 108)—add them 5 minutes into cooking the fresh cheese.

LAUKI SQUASH AND GREEN PAPAYA SOUP

PREP: 5 MINUTES ■ **COOK:** ABOUT 25 MINUTES   serves 4

This is an example of a warm dish that will cool down your body. The cooling and calming effect plus the soft texture of this soup feels like giving yourself a "food hug." Both lauki squash and green papaya (medium size is best) are sold in Indian and Asian grocery stores. Other names for pale-green lauki (*Lagenaria siceraria*): louki, bottle gourd, calabash, kaddu, doodhi, ghiya, opo.

4 cups peeled and cubed (1-inch cubes) lauki squash

1 cup peeled and cubed (½-inch cubes) green papaya

1 tablespoon olive oil

1½ teaspoons salt

6 curry leaves

1 teaspoon Cooling Masala (page 221)

½ teaspoon ground cumin

GARNISHES

2 tablespoons minced fresh dill

2 teaspoons fresh lime juice, or to taste

FOR AIRY DIGESTION: Substitute Digestive Masala (page 223) for the Cooling Masala.

FOR EARTHY DIGESTION: Add 1 teaspoon grated fresh ginger in Step 1.

1. In a 2- to 3-quart pot, combine the squash and papaya with 3 cups water. Add the olive oil, salt, curry leaves, masala, and cumin; cover and bring to a boil over medium-high heat.

2. Reduce the heat to low and simmer for about 15 minutes, until the vegetables are cooked to translucent tenderness.

3. Remove from the heat, uncover, and let the soup cool for at least 5 minutes. The soup may look unappealing to you at this point, but wait until you blend it!

4. Blend until smooth; add more water if needed to thin it.

5. Garnish with fresh dill and lime juice. Serve hot or warm.

NOTES

■ If you can't find lauki squash, use yellow squash or zucchini instead.

■ If you can't find green papaya, use the same amount of daikon radish. This combination is good for the kidneys.

The Healing Benefits of Lauki Squash

Much loved in Ayurveda, lauki squash is one of the best and oldest vegetables on the planet. It is light to digest, nourishes every body tissue, and acts as a "peace-maker" among the five elements. With its sweet and astringent taste, lauki squash cools down excessive overall heat, especially an overheated liver. Unlike other watery squashes, lauki squash will not imbalance the Earthy, who have a tendency to retain water. On a more subtle level, lauki is said to open the heart and calm the emotions. Ayurveda highly recommends lauki for pregnant women.

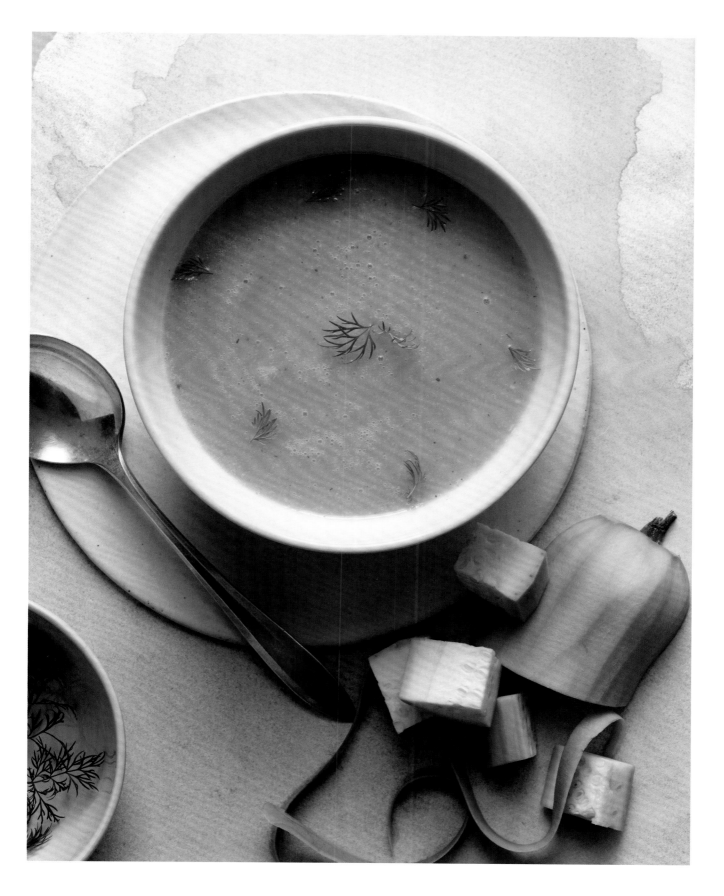

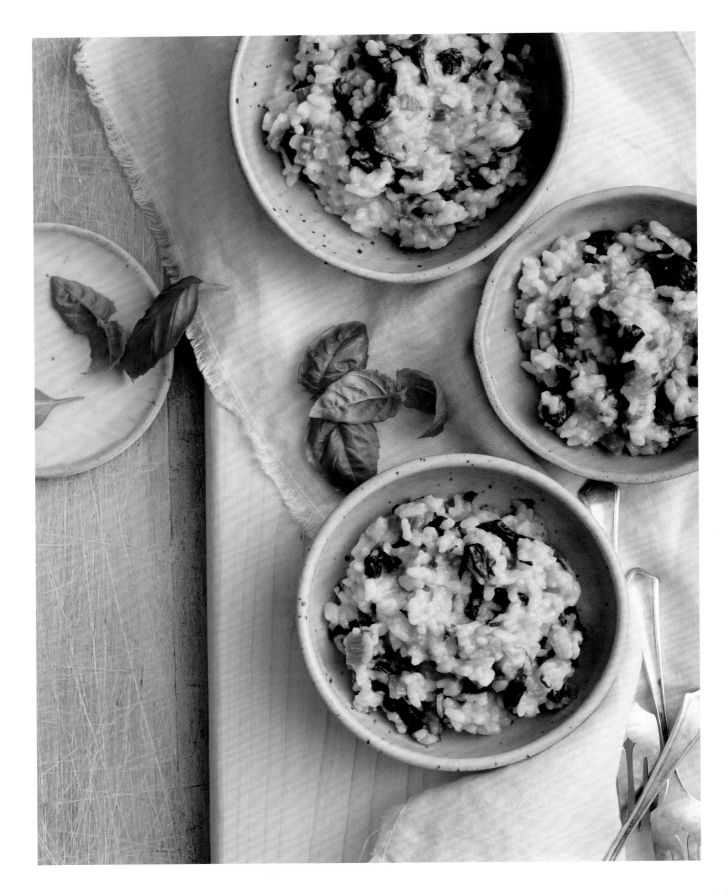

SPINACH RISOTTO

PREP: 5 MINUTES ■ **COOK:** ABOUT 45 MINUTES   serves 4 `GF` `DF`

This recipe lets us apply Ayurveda to north Italian cuisine! Although Arborio rice is much starchier than basmati rice and not traditional to Indian Ayurvedic dishes, it should not create heavy discomfort for someone with sharp Fiery digestion.

Frequent but not constant stirring is necessary to produce the creamy texture characteristic of risotto. This dish does require your attention, but it is not an all-consuming culinary feat—you can tackle small tasks in between stirs. As you patiently ladle broth into the sautéed rice, the grains become soft and slightly chewy, swimming in creamy sauce. Vegetable stock creates a delicate flavor foundation and is an essential ingredient for almost any risotto.

Risotto upgrades rice to a satisfying main course with some vegetables on the side. For an Italian-style meal, serve Spinach Risotto (page 111) with Kale and Arugula Pesto (page 190) and a colorful salad.

4½ to 5 cups Winter Vegetable Stock variation for Fiery Digestion (page 161) or water

1 tablespoon ghee or olive oil

⅛ teaspoon asafoetida (optional)

1 cup minced fennel or celery

1 cup medium-grain risotto rice (Vialone Nano, Carnaroli, or Arborio are best), rinsed

1 teaspoon ground coriander

3 cups packed spinach leaves

2 tablespoons minced fresh parsley leaves

2 tablespoons minced fresh basil leaves

1 teaspoon salt, or to taste

¼ teaspoon freshly ground black pepper (omit if you have acidic digestion)

1 tablespoon fresh lime juice

1 teaspoon olive oil

FOR AIRY DIGESTION: Enjoy as is.

FOR EARTHY DIGESTION: This dish might be too heavy for you, so taste a small serving.

1. Bring the stock to a simmer in a medium saucepan; keep it warm over low heat.

2. Heat the ghee in a 3- to 4-quart heavy-bottomed saucepan or sauté pan over medium heat. Add the asafoetida, if using, and the fennel and sauté until translucent and lightly golden, about 5 minutes. Using a wooden spatula or spoon, stir in the rice and coriander and sauté for 1 minute.

3. Reduce the heat to low, add 1 cup of the warm stock, and cook, stirring frequently until the rice soaks up the liquid. Continue cooking by adding stock in ½-cup increments, stirring every minute or two for about 10 seconds, until the rice is almost fully cooked, about 20 minutes.

4. Fold in the spinach, parsley, and basil and continue cooking (add more stock if needed) until the rice is creamy and soft but still a bit chewy, about 5 minutes.

5. Remove the pot from the heat and energetically stir in the salt, pepper, and lime juice. Drizzle with the oil and serve immediately.

LASAGNA WITH BROCCOLINI, CARROTS, AND SPINACH

PREP: 30 MINUTES (WITH ALREADY MADE BÉCHAMEL
AND FRESH SOFT CHEESE) ▪ **COOK:** 20 MINUTES

serves 6

This is my "Ayurvedized" version of this famous Italian dish. Alternate layers of colorful vegetables make this lasagna especially attractive. I've served it to from four to one hundred guests at Bhagavat Life at once, and a frequent and very gratifying comment I receive is "I can't believe how light your lasagna feels in my stomach!" I am certain that the almond milk béchamel, whole-grain noodles, and fresh cheeses make this lasagna rich yet much lighter and easier to digest without compromising appearance, taste, or flavor.

Making lasagna is like constructing a house, with the lasagna noodles as the foundation and the sauce as the plaster at each level. It takes time and patience, so plan ahead. You can make the soft fresh cheese and almond milk for the béchamel and grate the mozzarella the day before. It is worth all the effort, and I guarantee you that this dish will please friends and family (and kids!) on special occasions.

Serve it with Kale and Arugula Pesto (page 190) and a light salad.

3½ tablespoons ghee or olive oil

¼ teaspoon asafoetida (optional)

½ pound carrots, peeled and cut into
¼-inch slices (about 1½ cups)

1½ teaspoons salt

¼ teaspoon freshly ground black pepper

4 cups Almond Milk Béchamel Sauce
(double the recipe on page 188)

12 ounces broccolini or broccoli

1½ cups fresh soft cheese (page 202),
crumbled and mixed with ½ teaspoon salt

½ pound baby spinach, chopped

1 pound whole-grain lasagna sheets
(wheat or gluten-free)

1 cup grated fresh mozzarella cheese

FOR AIRY DIGESTION: Enjoy as it is with some Grounding Digestive Tea (page 180) after your meal.

FOR EARTHY DIGESTION: This dish is too heavy for you, so be happy with a smaller portion and a few extra turns of cracked black pepper on top. Chew on some Earthy digestive spice blend (page 51) after your meal.

1. Heat 1½ tablespoons of the ghee in a skillet over medium-low heat. Add the asafoetida, if using, and the carrots and sauté, stirring occasionally, until the carrots are tender and lightly colored but not mushy, about 10 minutes. Set aside in a bowl and season with ½ teaspoon of the salt, the black pepper, and ¾ cup of the béchamel.

2. Bring 3 quarts of water to a boil in a large pot. Remove and discard the ends of the broccolini stalks. Cut the tops into larger florets, for about 4 cups stems and florets. When the water comes to a boil, add the remaining

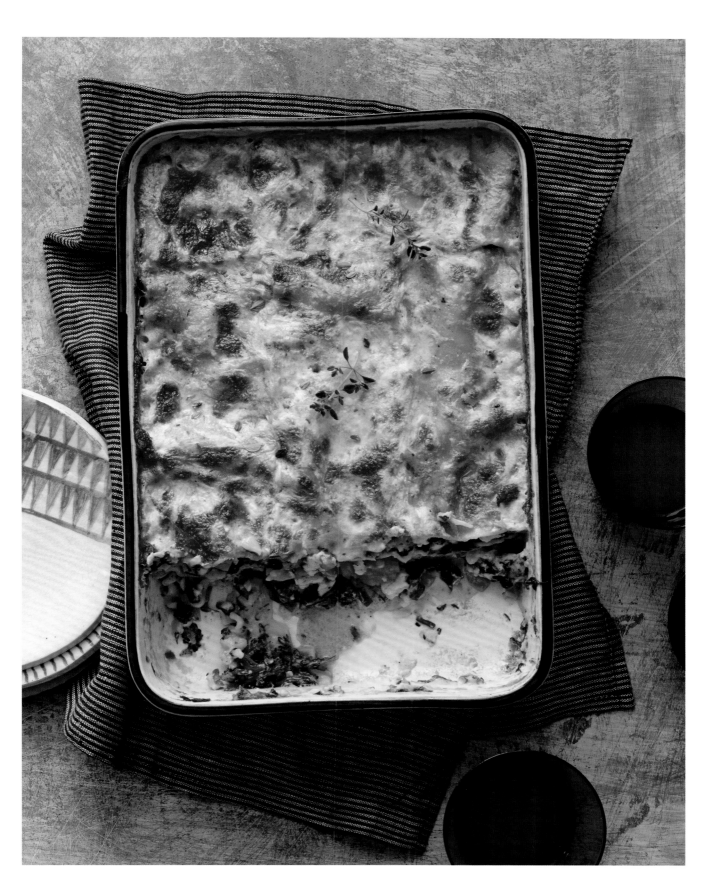

1 teaspoon salt and the broccolini and cook for 2 minutes. Spoon out the broccolini (reserve the cooking water for cooking the noodles), refresh it under cold running water, and drain well. Cut the stalks and the florets into ¼-inch pieces.

3. Melt 1 tablespoon of the ghee in a clean skillet. Add the broccolini, and 1 tablespoon water. Cook the broccolini uncovered, stirring occasionally, until tender but not mushy, about 3 minutes. Set aside in a separate bowl and mix in ¾ cup of the remaining béchamel.

4. Bring the water from cooking the broccolini back to a boil and add the lasagna noodles. Cook according to the package instructions, then transfer them to a wide bowl of cold water.

5. Preheat the oven to 350'F.

6. Grease a 9 x 13-inch lasagna pan with the remaining tablespoon ghee or olive oil.

7. Smear 3 tablespoons of béchamel across the bottom of the pan. Line the pan with a layer of lasagna noodles. If needed, cut the noodles so they touch but do not overlap. Evenly spread the broccolini mixture over the noodles, making sure the noodles are well coated with béchamel. Sprinkle ½ cup of the fresh soft cheese on top. Cover with another layer of noodles and repeat the process, using the carrot mixture and ½ cup fresh soft cheese as the second layer. Make a third layer with noodles, spinach, and ½ cup fresh soft cheese. Top that with a final layer of noodles, coating them with the remaining béchamel, then sprinkle with the mozzarella.

8. Bake the lasagna until the top turns golden brown in spots and the sauce is bubbling, about 20 minutes. Let it stand for 5 minutes, then cut into squares and serve immediately.

VARIATION

■ **Dairy-free option:** Replace the two cheeses with 2 cups cashews soaked overnight, drained, and pulsed in a food processor with 1 teaspoon salt and a little water to a ricotta-like consistency.

BROCCOLI WITH FRESH CHEESE

PREP: 5 MINUTES (WITH ALREADY MADE PRESSED CHEESE) ■
COOK: 10 MINUTES

serves 4 `GF` `DF`

All cruciferous vegetables, including broccoli, are best eaten with proteins. Broccoli is high in nutrients and low in calories and is especially balancing for when you're feeling Fiery or Earthy. Broccoli with Fresh Cheese is a particularly satisfying dish. Its mild flavors and appealing looks exemplify greatness in simplicity. For a quick meal, serve with Basmati Rice and Red Quinoa (page 101) and Cilantro Chutney (page 191).

4 cups chopped (1-inch florets) broccoli

1¾ teaspoons salt

2 teaspoons ghee or olive oil

1 tablespoon olive oil

½ teaspoon cumin seeds

1 teaspoon grated fresh ginger

⅛ teaspoon asafoetida (omit if you have acidic digestion)

¼ teaspoon freshly ground black pepper (omit if you have acidic digestion)

1 cup cubed (1-inch cubes) fresh pressed cheese (page 202; omit for dairy-free option)

GARNISH

Lime slices

FOR AIRY DIGESTION: Add a second teaspoon of ginger in Step 2.

FOR EARTHY DIGESTION: Reduce the cheese or replace it with 1 extra cup chopped broccoli or cauliflower; add 1 seeded and minced small green Thai chile with the ginger in Step 2.

1. In a 3-quart saucepan, bring 6 cups water to a boil and add 1 teaspoon salt. Add the broccoli and cook until it is soft and vibrant green, 4 to 5 minutes. Drain the broccoli and rinse with cold water; set aside to drain. Alternatively, you may steam the broccoli—in this case, omit the initial 1 teaspoon salt. (You may save the broccoli water to cook grains or soups.)

2. In a medium heavy skillet, heat the ghee and olive oil over medium-low heat; add the cumin seeds and cook for 5 to 10 seconds, until the cumin releases its aroma. Add the ginger and cook for 5 to 10 seconds more. Quickly follow with asafoetida, black pepper, the remaining ¾ teaspoon salt, the broccoli, and cheese cubes. Add 2 tablespoons water, increase the heat to medium-high, and stir-fry with a metal spatula for about 5 minutes to allow the vegetables and cheese to absorb the seasonings and moisture, until the broccoli is tender. Be careful to not mash the broccoli.

3. Serve hot with lime slices.

VARIATION

■ Substitute Golden Cheese Cubes (page 193) for the plain cheese cubes.

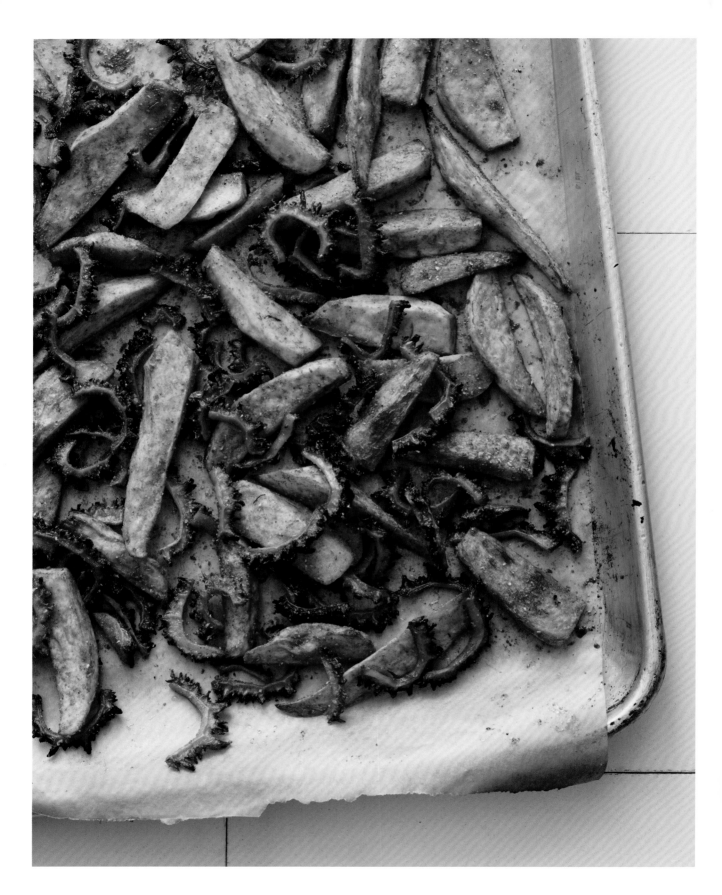

BITTER MELON AND TARO "FRIES"

PREP: 10 TO 15 MINUTES ▪ **COOK:** ABOUT 20 MINUTES   serves 3 to 4 `GF` `DF`

Even if bitter is your least favorite taste, it is still superb for reducing the accumulation of Fiery and Earthy energies, though it can increase the movement of our bodily airs. Taro root adds sweetness and balances our airiness. If you enjoy bitter melon straight, go for it and substitute it for the taro. Serve Bitter Melon and Taro "Fries" as a side dish to sweeter vegetables or grains with some Cilantro Chutney (page 191) or Raisin-Cranberry Sauce (page 189).

2 medium Indian bitter melons
   (about ½ pound)

3 medium taro roots

1 teaspoon ground coriander

½ teaspoon Cooling Masala (page 221)

¼ teaspoon ground turmeric

½ teaspoon salt

2 tablespoons melted ghee or coconut oil

GARNISH

Lime slices

> **FOR AIRY DIGESTION:** Replace one of the bitter melons with one or two additional taros.
>
> **FOR EARTHY DIGESTION:** Substitute Energizing Masala (page 221) for the Cooling Masala.

1. Preheat the oven to 400°F.

2. Wash and pat-dry the bitter melons. Cut off the ends and cut in half lengthwise. Scoop out the seeds with a small spoon to create "boats." Slice each boat across into ¼-inch pieces (about 2 cups). Peel the taro root, cut it into ½-inch-thick fry shapes (about 1½ cups), rinse, and pat-dry.

3. Lay the vegetables on a baking sheet and sprinkle with the coriander, masala, turmeric, and salt; drizzle with the ghee and use your hands to rub everything into the vegetables. Roast, stirring occasionally, until the they are crispy with a golden crust, about 20 minutes.

4. Garnish each serving with a squeeze of lime. It will counteract some of the bitterness.

The Healing Benefits of Bitter Melon

Including bitter melon in our diets is important because of its high nutritional value and powerful detoxifying properties. Here are some of its benefits:

- Cleanses the liver and pancreas, purifies the blood, and improves blood circulation

- Lowers blood sugar and hypertension

- Enhances digestion

- Reduces inflammation

- High in phosphorus, manganese, magnesium, and zinc; vitamins B1, B2, B3, and C; thiamine, foliate, and riboflavin

Caution: Do not eat bitter melon excessively and never eat it raw, as it may lead to severe digestive problems. Avoid consuming it during pregnancy and while breast-feeding.

SAUTÉED LEAFY GREENS

PREP: 5 TO 10 MINUTES ▪ **COOK:** 5 MINUTES   serves 4 `GF` `DF`

I was fortunate to take an Ayurvedic cooking training with Dr. Shanti Kumar Kamlesh, a Vaidya who teaches at Sivananda Yoga Ashrams around the world. One thing he said always stuck with me: "We need to eat something green every day. Whenever you plan a meal, think 'a quarter green.'" What "green" did you have today?

Greens including leafy greens, fresh herbs, broccoli, cabbage, green beans, bok choy, and asparagus are rich in minerals, chlorophyll, and fiber and are an excellent detox food for the liver, colon, and blood. Greens tend to be of an Airy, cooling, and bitter nature, and to enjoy them without any gassy or bloating reactions, it is best to lightly steam or sauté them. These cooking methods will protect most of the nutrients, ease digestion, and neutralize harmful chemical compounds such as oxalates and phytates found in most leafy greens.

Slightly bitter Sautéed Leafy Greens go well with any cheese, grain, lentil, or vegetable dish.

2 tablespoons ghee or coconut oil

½ teaspoon fenugreek seeds

½ teaspoon Superspice Masala (page 219) or Digestive Masala (page 223)

12 cups stemmed and chopped (1-inch strips) leafy greens such as chard, beet greens, collards, spinach, and/or kale (about 1 pound)

¾ teaspoon salt

GARNISHES

Pinch of freshly ground black pepper (optional)

Fresh lime juice

FOR AIRY DIGESTION: Add 2 teaspoons grated fresh ginger at the end of toasting the fenugreek seeds in Step 1. Drizzle a little olive oil in Step 3 just before serving.

FOR EARTHY DIGESTION: Reduce the oil to 2 teaspoons in Step 1 and add 2 teaspoons grated fresh ginger and 1 seeded and minced small green Thai chile at the end of toasting the fenugreek seeds.

1. Heat the ghee in a large skillet or wok over low heat. Add the fenugreek seeds and cook until the seeds turn dark brown, about 2 minutes.

2. Add the masala followed immediately by the leafy greens. If the greens do not fit in the skillet, add them in batches, using salad tongs to tuck the fresh leaves under the wilted ones. Cover the pot for only a minute to let the greens wilt and shrink. Continue to sauté, turning the greens frequently until they are tender yet still vibrant green, 4 to 5 minutes. Be careful not to overcook them.

3. Turn off the heat and leave the greens uncovered to cool for a minute. Add the salt and serve immediately, garnished with the pepper and lime juice.

RAW SALAD COMBINATIONS FOR THE SUMMER

PREP: 5 TO 15 MINUTES ▪ **ASSEMBLE:** 5 MINUTES   GF DF

If your digestion is strong enough for raw food, you can make your own salad bowl and top it with any of the salad dressings on pages 196 to 199. These are just a few suggestions. In general, avoid mixing raw vegetables and fruits together, as they are almost always incompatible for digestion. For more protein, you can add nuts or seeds (soaked or toasted)—sunflower seeds, almonds, walnuts, pecans—or fresh cheese cubes (page 202) to any leafy green salad.

1. Arugula, red radish, celery

2. Romaine and red leaf lettuce, cucumber, nasturtium flowers or yellow endive

3. Avocado, snow peas, red radish, watercress

4. Spring mix, grated carrots, cucumbers

5. Spiralized noodles from zucchini, yellow squash, daikon radish, kohlrabi, cucumber, carrot, red radish with chopped avocado and pistachios.

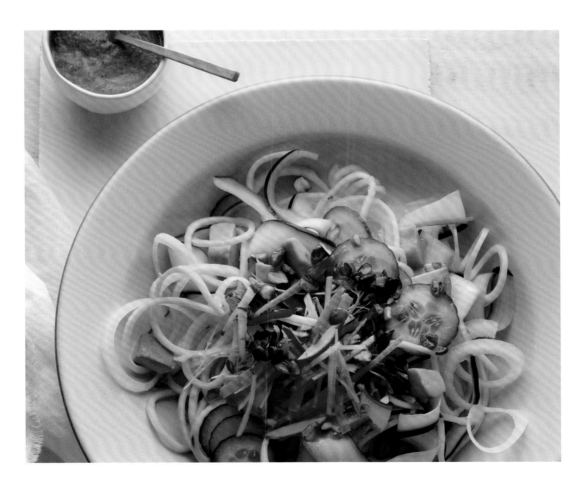

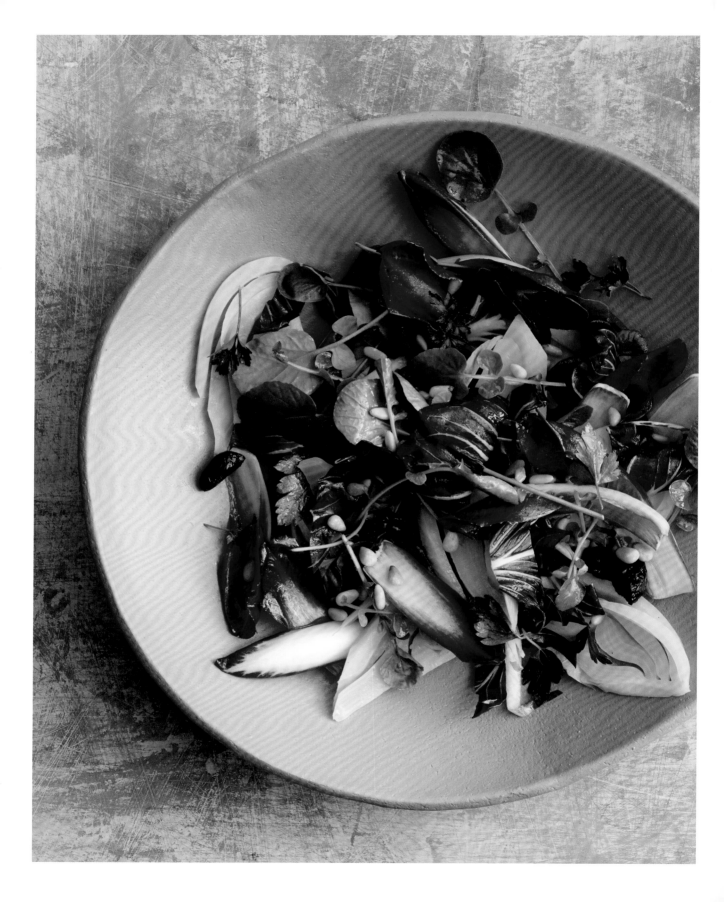

FENNEL, RADICCHIO, AND WATERCRESS SALAD

PREP: 10 MINUTES ▪ **COOK:** 10 MINUTES

serves 4 **GF** **DF**

Radicchio lettuce, with its beautiful red and purple leaves and pleasantly bitter taste, is actually Italian chicory, and it is also known as red endive or red chicory. You can use any radicchio variety for this salad.

The pale green fennel, darker green watercress, and magenta-colored radicchio contrast in color and complement each other with their sweet, astringent, and bitter tastes—all so balancing in the summer.

3 small fennel bulbs

1 small radicchio, leaves separated, rinsed, drained, and coarsely chopped (about 1 cup)

1 bunch watercress, washed, drained, and coarsely chopped (about 2 cups)

2 tablespoons pitted and halved black olives

2 tablespoons chopped fresh basil, parsley, or dill

2 tablespoons lightly toasted pine nuts

DRESSING

¼ cup olive oil

2 tablespoons fresh lime juice

2 tablespoons fresh orange juice

½ teaspoon salt

Pinch of freshly ground black pepper

FOR AIRY DIGESTION: Omit the radicchio.

FOR EARTHY DIGESTION: Add 1 tablespoon ginger juice to the dressing in Step 4.

1. Remove the tops of the fennel bulbs and cut off the base and any outer bruised leaves. Quarter each bulb and cut out the hard core. Cut the fennel into ¼-inch wedges (about 3 cups).

2. In a steamer, steam the fennel until it is soft and translucent, 5 minutes. Refresh it in a bowl of ice-cold water, then drain well immediately.

3. Toss the fennel, radicchio, watercress, olives, and basil in a bowl; sprinkle the pine nuts on top.

4. To make the dressing, whisk the oil, lime juice, orange juice, salt, and pepper in a small bowl. Spoon the dressing over the salad, toss gently, and serve immediately.

VARIATIONS

▪ Substitute 2 cups baby arugula for the watercress.

▪ Substitute 2 yellow endives for the radicchio.

▪ Keep the fennel raw, but slice it very thin (ideally with a mandoline).

▪ Add 1 cup fresh pressed cheese cubes (page 202) in Step 3.

▪ Reserve 4 smaller radicchio leaves and fill them with salad for individual servings.

STUFFED AVOCADOS WITH FRESH CHEESE

PREP: ABOUT 20 MINUTES (WITH ALREADY MADE FRESH CHEESE)   *serves 6* GF

I created this recipe during my recovery from a long, stressful period, when I ended up under-weight and with very dry skin (the symptoms of prolonged Airy imbalance). I had to eat a diet of grounding foods that are a bit heavier, warm, moist, and fatty. Healthy fats, protein, potassium, omega-3 fatty acids—Stuffed Avocados with Fresh Cheese has all of them in abundance. The spices and fresh herbs here are a must for digestion. I will be straight with you: this recipe is for those who crave protein or want to gain weight, not lose it. It is also perfect for pregnant and nursing mothers, and most kids will love it.

The crunchy celery and walnuts contrast with the creamy, fatty avocados and cheese, while leaving room for the olives to make their flavor statement. You may serve Stuffed Avocados with Fresh Cheese as a succulent appetizer or a side for lunch. It is also good as a protein snack in late morning. Eat it at night only if you experience the insatiable appetite of sharp Fiery digestion.

3 ripe Haas avocados

½ fresh lime

1 cup fresh soft cheese (page 202)

¼ cup minced celery

3 tablespoons minced fresh basil leaves

2 tablespoons pitted and minced black olives

1 tablespoon minced fresh parsley leaves

½ teaspoon freshly ground black pepper
 (omit if you have acidic stomach)

¼ teaspoon salt

¼ teaspoon black salt

GARNISHES

¼ cup finely chopped walnuts

6 whole parsley leaves (optional)

FOR AIRY DIGESTION: Add an extra ¼ tea-spoon ground black pepper in Step 3.

FOR EARTHY DIGESTION: This recipe is not for you today. If you still want to go for it, chew a few slices of fresh ginger before enjoying it. You may also sprinkle extra black pepper on top or serve with a teaspoon of spicy pickle.

1. Cut the avocados in half lengthwise and remove the pit from each. Do not peel the avocados.

2. Using a small spoon, make an avocado boat by scooping out part of the avocado meat, leaving a ¼-inch border lining the skin. Chop or mash the scooped avocado and transfer it to a mixing bowl. Sprinkle the avocado boats and chopped pulp with a little bit of fresh lime juice—this will prevent them from browning.

3. To the mashed avocado, add the cheese (make sure there are no big lumps), celery, basil, olives, parsley, black pepper, salt, and black salt. Use your loving hands to mix and mash everything into a chunky filling.

4. Heap each avocado boat with the filling.

5. Garnish each stuffed avocado with walnuts and a parsley leaf. Serve at room temperature.

6. To store, cover and refrigerate for up to a day. Take the stuffed avocados out of the refrigerator at least 30 minutes before serving.

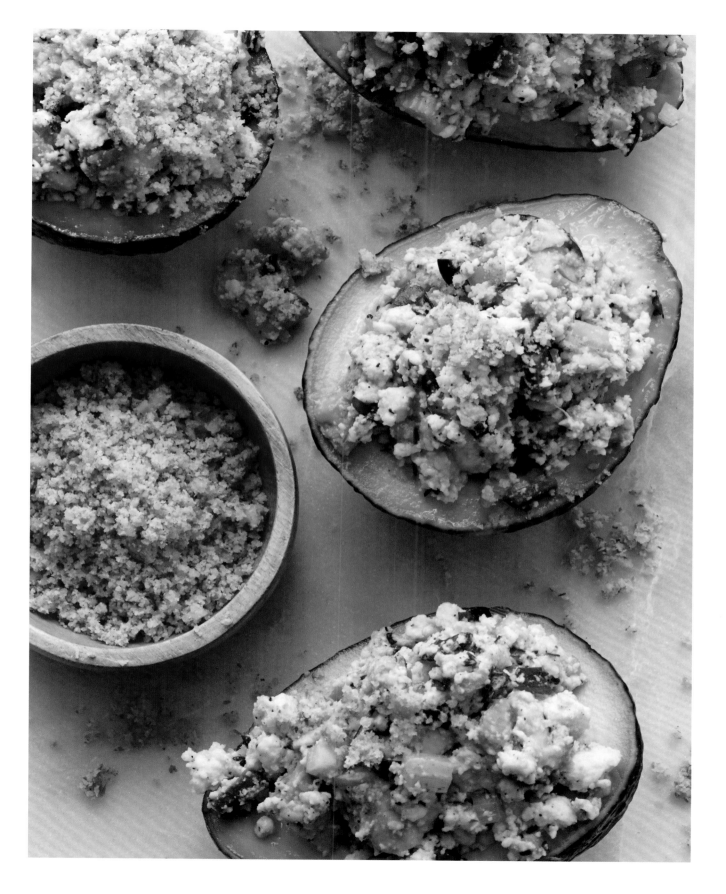

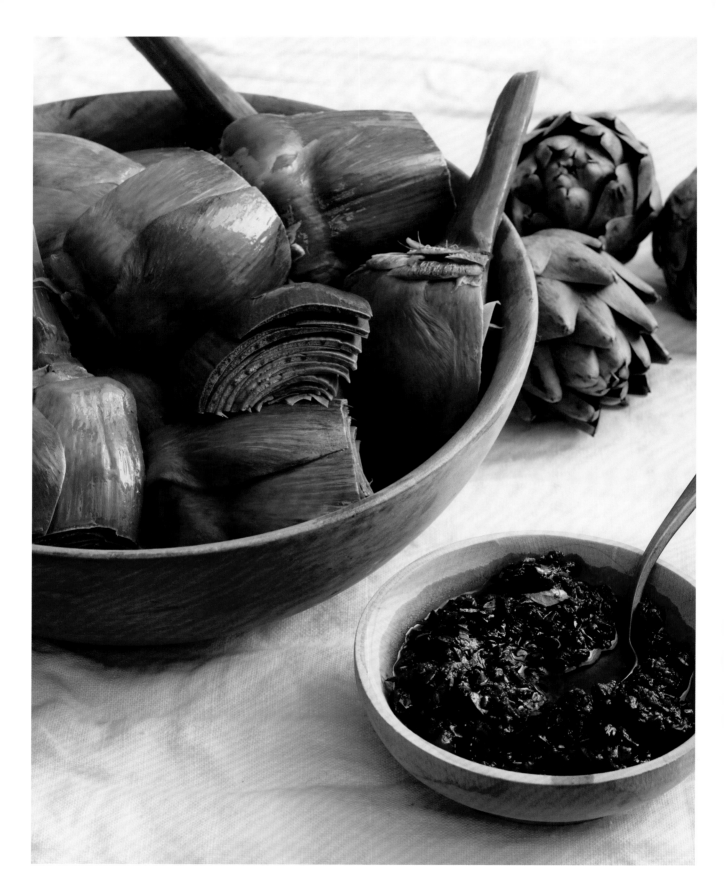

STEAMED ARTICHOKES WITH OLIVE TAPENADE

PREP: 10 MINUTES ▪ **COOK:** ABOUT 30 MINUTES

serves 4 GF DF

I love watching guests trying to eat an artichoke for the first time. They turn it around, look at it suspiciously from all sides, smell it, and try biting at it, until they give up and ask, "How do you eat this thing?" I show them how to pull off an outer petal, pull it through the teeth to remove the soft pulp and discard the rest; then move on to the next petal until we reach the best part: the heart. "That's a lot of work and a lot of waste!" my guests would exclaim, gazing at the pile of inedible fiber. Yes, it takes work to reach to the heart of anything (or anyone).

Steamed Artichokes with Olive Tapenade can be served hot or at room temperature with another dip or sauce such as Kale and Arugula Pesto (page 190) or Sunflower-Sesame Dip (page 197). They go well with Spinach Risotto (page 111) and Fennel, Radicchio, and Watercress Salad (page 121).

4 medium artichokes (about 2 pounds), rinsed

1 lime, cut in half

3 bay leaves

Salt

TAPENADE

1 tablespoon olive oil

⅛ teaspoon asafoetida (omit if you have acidic digestion)

¼ teaspoon freshly ground black pepper (omit if you have acidic digestion)

⅓ cup black olives, pitted and coarsely chopped

2 tablespoons fresh lime juice

2 tablespoons minced fresh parsley leaves

2 tablespoons chopped fresh basil leaves

1 tablespoon chopped fresh mint leaves

1 teaspoon fresh lemon thyme leaves (optional)

FOR AIRY DIGESTION: Add more lime juice and pepper to taste.

FOR EARTHY DIGESTION: These might be a bit too heavy for your slow digestion, so eat a smaller portion. Reduce the olive oil to 2 teaspoons; add more pepper to taste.

1. Working one artichoke at a time, snap off several layers of the tough outer leaves until you reach the leaves that are mostly pale green. With a sharp knife or scissors, cut the artichoke leaves across to remove the prickly tips. Trim the end of the stem and peel the stem's outer layer with a vegetable peeler. Use a lime half to rub juice on the trimmed parts of the artichoke to protect them from oxidizing. Quarter the artichoke lengthwise (leave the stem attached). With a small spoon or a paring knife, scoop out the fuzzy choke in the middle and discard it. Rub some more lime on the freshly cut artichoke pieces.

2. Set a steamer over boiling water and add the bay leaves to the water. Sprinkle salt over the artichokes and steam them until they are quite tender and the outer leaves pull off easily, 20 to 25 minutes.

3. While the artichokes are cooking, prepare the dressing. Lightly heat the olive oil with the asafoetida and black pepper, if using, in a metal measuring cup or a small pan, not more than 10 seconds. Remove from the heat and set aside.

4. In a small chopper or blender, pulse the olives and lime juice to a minced chunky consistency; add the infused olive oil and the fresh herbs and pulse a couple more times to incorporate them.

5. Serve the cooked artichokes warm, with the olive tapenade on the side.

NOTE

- For baby artichokes, use 8 to 10; follow the same trimming instructions but cut them in half rather than quarters.

The Healing Benefits of Artichokes

With their astringent and sweet tastes and heavy qualities, artichokes are very filling and satisfying for a Fiery person with strong appetite. They are an alkalizing food and are suitable to include in weight reduction or diabetic diets. Here are some more benefits:

- Strengthen the functions of the liver and gallbladder
- High in cynarin, which increases bile production and thus fat assimilation
- High in glutathione and other antioxidants
- Have diuretic qualities
- Reduce cholesterol
- Rich in vitamins A and C (to help fight off infection)
- High in calcium and iron

Caution: Avoid eating artichokes if you suffer from inflammation of the bowel.

COCONUT PAPAYA SMOOTHIE

PREP: 5 MINUTES (WITH ALREADY PREPARED COCONUT MILK)   serves 2 (makes 16 ounces) GF DF

Unique flavor unfolds when you add maple syrup to papaya and coconut—no other sweetener can match it. For me it was love at first taste. This soft-orange smoothie is best served alone as a late-morning or afternoon snack on a hot summer day. If your digestive fire is ablaze in the morning, then have it for breakfast.

2 cups peeled, seeded, and chopped papaya
1 cup coconut milk (page 217)
¾ cup coconut water or filtered water
3 tablespoons maple syrup, or to taste
Small pinch of ground cardamom seeds

Combine all the ingredients in a blender and blend until smooth. Adjust the water and sweetener, if you like. To store, refrigerate in a jar or closed container for up to 24 hours. Enjoy at room temperature.

NOTES

■ Shop for very ripe and soft papaya, preferably non-GMO. If after making the smoothie you have some left, eat it at lunchtime as a digestive aid.

The Healing Benefits of Coconut

Coconut is highly nutritious and rich in fiber, good fats, vitamins, and minerals. From an Ayurvedic point of view, coconut is sweet, heavy, fatty, and cooling and is most balancing for the Fiery and the Airy (in summer). If you experience symptoms of Earthy imbalance, such as weight gain, congestion, bronchitis, or poor circulation, then it is best to reduce the consumption of coconut products until you restore your balance.

Because coconut is so cooling, summer is the best season to enjoy it. Drinking a glass of fresh coconut water in the morning will help your body withstand heat.

These are just a few of the benefits of coconut described by ancient and modern researchers:

■ Prevents heart disease

■ Nourishes the brain

■ Balances blood sugar

■ Enhances the immune system

■ Promotes healthy hair and complexion

■ Has antibacterial and antiviral properties

■ Relieves and eliminates hemorrhoids

ALMOND ROSE DELIGHT

SOAK: AT LEAST 12 HOURS FOR THE ALMONDS; 15 MINUTES FOR THE AGAR AGAR ▪
PREP: 10 TO 15 MINUTES ▪ **COOK:** ABOUT 5 MINUTES ▪ **CHILL:** AT LEAST 1 HOUR ▪ serves 8 to 10 GF DF

Soft and delicate, fragrant and beautiful—the famed qualities of rose remain intact with the flan-like texture, aromatic taste, and pleasing appearance of this dessert. The combination of ingredients may seem unusual, but trust me, as soon as you take a bite and let it linger in your mouth, within seconds "May I have another one?" will follow.

Everything rose—be it as flower, perfume, oil, water, or tea—is your best friend when you need to calm down, chill out, or speak with an open heart. Go to page 130 to learn more about the healing benefits of rose.

Agar agar flakes are available in health food stores and Asian grocery stores. I like the Eden brand. Many thanks to my dear friend and cooking mentor Kandarpa Bhuckory for sharing this recipe.

3 tablespoons agar agar flakes or
  2 tablespoons agar agar powder
  (see note page 130)

¾ cup raw almonds, soaked in water for at
  least 12 hours or overnight, rinsed and
  drained

½ cup plus 1 tablespoon raw cane sugar
  (choose a lighter color)

¼ teaspoon ground cardamom seeds

2 tablespoons food-grade rose water

1 teaspoon crushed dried rose petals or
  rose buds

FOR AIRY DIGESTION: Enjoy it as is; it's best at room temperature.

FOR EARTHY DIGESTION: Try a piece, but remember that it's best for you to cut down on sweets.

---

1. In a 1- to 2-quart skillet or saucepan, soak the agar agar flakes in 1 cup filtered water for 20 minutes (10 minutes for agar agar powder).

2. In the meantime, place the almonds in a heatproof bowl. Blanch them by covering them with 1½ cups boiling hot water for 7 seconds. Drain immediately and rinse. Seven seconds of blanching will keep the almonds "alive" yet easy to skin. Practice patience and peel all of the almonds—this step is important for texture, appearance, and your peace of mind.

3. Place the peeled almonds in a blender with 1¼ cups water and blend until very smooth. (A blender on high speed works best here, better than a food processor or an electric chopper.)

4. Bring the soaked agar agar to a boil. Stir almost constantly for 5 to 7 minutes, until the flakes have dissolved completely and turn into a gelatinous liquid. Add the sugar and

OPPOSITE: Almond Rose Delight, Heart-Opening Tea

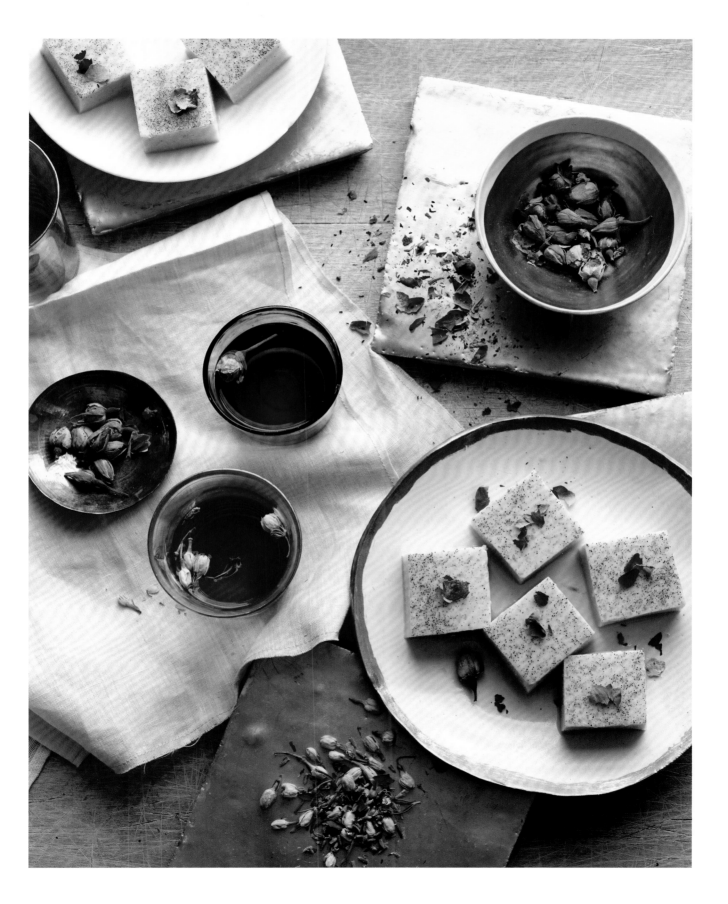

stir to dissolve it. Turn off the heat and set aside for a minute.

5. Add the blended almonds, cardamom, and rose water to the hot agar–sugar mixture and mix well.

6. Pour into individual small bowls or a small dish (a square 8-inch Pyrex dish works great) to a 1-inch thickness. Refrigerate for at least 1 hour, until thick and cool.

7. Cut into 2-inch square pieces, turn them upside down, and garnish with the crushed dried rose petals.

8. To store, cover and refrigerate for up to 3 days.

NOTES

- Agar agar is a seaweed used as a gelatin substitute (gelatin is not vegetarian). It is very soothing to the stomach and rich in minerals and has mild detox properties.

- I find raw cane sugar to be the best sweetener for this dessert. Coconut sugar's darker color and strong taste will overpower the delicate rose water. You also could omit the raw sugar and serve individual pieces with a drizzle of maple syrup.

Giving Your Skin a Healthy Glow with Rose Water

Rose water (aka rose hydrosol) is the by-product of the distillation of rose petals during the production of rose oil. For centuries, rose water has been used in beauty care to tone and hydrate the skin and to maintain the skin's radiance and youthfulness. It is also an instant mood lifter when you're feeling worn down, depressed, or angry or you are grieving. I keep a small bottle of rose water in my kitchen, bathroom, and travel bag. Here is how you can use it on your skin:

- As a skin toner, spray on every part of your body but especially your face and neck after cleansing, washing off a facial mask, or before applying nourishing oil or cream.

- Dab rose water with cotton balls on your face to balance the skin, open blocked pores, restore radiance to your complexion, and prevent wrinkles.

- If you work a lot on a computer, your eyes and face can become dry and dull from the heating electromagnetic frequencies. Stop for a minute every hour and spray your face with a few spritzes of rose water. So refreshing!

- Air travel and airplane air are very drying and depleting for the skin. Carry a small (2-ounce or less) spray bottle of rose water and spray your face every hour or so.

- For tired, irritated, or puffy eyes, moisten two cotton pads with cold rose water, place them on your eyes, lie down, and relax for 10 to 15 minutes.

LIME MOUSSE

SOAK: 8 HOURS OR OVERNIGHT ▪
PREP: ABOUT 15 MINUTES (WITH ALREADY MADE ALMOND MILK)

serves 6 GF DF

Years ago, I was hired to develop the vegan raw menu for the Bhakti Café in Manhattan. This is how I created this dessert, and although it did not make it on the menu, it is a summer favorite of many of my students and clients. The creamy sweet-sour texture of this mousse is so refreshing, much more cooling and nourishing than ice cream. Please keep in mind that this is a very rich dessert, so serve it in small portions.

Soaking the cashews makes them less acidic and easier to digest and contributes to the thick, creamy consistency of this sweet. Sunflower lecithin is a natural emulsifier, creating a mousse-like texture; it is available in health food stores.

1½ cups cashews, soaked for 8 hours or overnight, drained, and rinsed

¾ cup almond milk (page 216)

½ cup fresh lime juice

½ cup raw cane sugar

1½ teaspoons vanilla extract

½ teaspoon ground cardamom

1 tablespoon sunflower lecithin

¼ cup plus 2 tablespoons melted coconut oil

GARNISH

Very thin slices of lime

> **FOR AIRY DIGESTION:** Enjoy as it is, closer to room temperature (not too cold).
>
> **FOR EARTHY DIGESTION:** This dessert is too heavy for you. Taste a bite and enjoy the happiness of sharing the rest.

1. In a blender, combine the cashews, almond milk, lime juice, sugar, vanilla, and cardamom and blend until very smooth and creamy.

2. Add the lecithin and coconut oil and blend again until the oil and lecithin are well incorporated.

3. Pour into small mousse cups or bowls, filling them by half or two-thirds.

4. Cover and refrigerate for at least 6 hours or overnight for the mousse to set.

5. Decorate each cup with a thin slice of lime and some berries if you like. Serve chilled. To store, cover and refrigerate for up to 3 days.

HYDRATING DRINK

PREP: 5 MINUTES   serves 2 (makes 16 ounces) GF DF

My SV Ayurveda teacher, Vaidya R. K. Mishra, has spoken so much about the importance of this beverage that I had to give you the recipe. Most of us city dwellers tend to become dehydrated because we live in very dry environments, surrounded by electric devices, heaters, the sun, the cold, and the wind, or sometimes we just don't drink enough alkaline spring water.

   I call this drink the "Ayurvedic Gatorade"—next to fresh coconut water, it is one of the best electrolyte beverages to quench your thirst down to the cellular level. Toasted cumin and nutmeg support absorption, and Soma Salt adds minerals—do not omit these. This drink tastes perfect when all six tastes meddle on your palate without a single taste standing out. Although I've placed this recipe in the Cooling Recipes chapter, this drink is balancing for everyone, in every season. Sip it when working out or during your detox days before you feel thirsty to prevent dehydration.

⅛ teaspoon cumin seeds

2 cups spring water

1 tablespoon fresh lime juice

2 teaspoons chopped fresh mint or basil leaves

1 teaspoon raw sugar

2 small pinches Soma Salt (see page 46)

⅛ teaspoon ground nutmeg (optional)

1. Dry-toast the cumin seeds in a small skillet over medium-low heat for 1 minute, or until they release their aroma. Remove from the heat and crush them in a mortar or spice grinder.

2. In a blender, briefly blend all the ingredients and strain through a cheesecloth or nut milk bag. Serve at room temperature.

3. To store, refrigerate in a jar or closed container for up to 3 days.

ROSE TEAS

My mom lives in the valley of the world-famous Bulgarian rose fields. For a few weeks in May and June, the area steeps in the intoxicating sweet scent of *Rosa damascena* (Damascus rose), while patient men and women carefully cut the flowers one by one, to be sent to the distilleries the same day. The end of the picking season culminates with rose festivals all over the area. It's a great time to visit Bulgaria and experience its ancient traditions!

For centuries, the rose has been a symbol of love, beauty, and spirituality. In Ayurveda it is used extensively to balance the five elements and slow down aging.

I've collected the following rose tea recipes during my years of study of SV Ayurveda. Use unsprayed dried rose buds or petals; organic is best.

LIVER-COOLING ROSE TEA

PREP: ABOUT 10 MINUTES   serves 2 `GF` `DF`

This blend supports the natural detox functions of the liver, a hot organ that tends to overheat due to stress, environmental pollution, eating processed and artificial foods, drinking alcohol, taking drugs, and so on. It also relieves acidic digestion.

2 dried rose buds or 1 teaspoon rose petals

⅛ teaspoon (a small pinch) coriander seeds

⅛ teaspoon (a small pinch) fennel seeds

⅛ teaspoon (a small pinch) DGL powder (deglycerized licorice powder; available at www.chandika.com)

2 cups boiling hot spring water

Combine the rose petals coriander seeds, fennel seeds, and DGL powder in a teapot. Pour in the boiling water, cover and steep for 10 minutes. Strain and enjoy in the morning or around lunchtime or to relieve acidic digestion.

EYE CARE ROSE TEA

PREP: ABOUT 10 MINUTES

serves 2

This tea is superb for when your eyes are tired, itchy, burning, or dry from prolonged gazing at computer or TV screen, being out in the hot sun, crying, or wearing chemical makeup.

2 dry-toasted and ground cloves

2 dried rose buds or 1 teaspoon rose petals

1 teaspoon chopped fresh mint leaves

2 cups boiling hot spring water

Tiny pinch of salt

1 teaspoon Sucanat or raw sugar (optional)

Combine the cloves, rose buds, and mint in a teapot. Pour in the boiling water, cover, and steep for 5 minutes. Strain and add the salt and sugar. Sip slowly throughout the day.

HEART-OPENING ROSE TEA

PREP: 7 MINUTES ■ **COOK:** 7 MINUTES

serves 2

This blend is amazing for when you feel heartbroken, negative, overcome by grief, or when you want to tell your restless mind "Shut up!" Organic dried rose buds or petals, lavender, and jasmine flowers are available at a few online stores. My favorite are www.chandika.com and www.mountainroseherbs.com.

2 cups spring water

4 dried rose buds or 2 teaspoons rose petals

½ teaspoon dried lavender flowers

3 dried jasmine flowers

In a small pot, bring the water to a boil. Add the rose buds and lavender, reduce the heat, cover, and simmer for 7 minutes. Turn off the heat, add the jasmine flowers, cover again, and steep for 7 more minutes. Strain and sip slowly.

The Healing Benefits of Rose (*Rosa damascena*)

- Soothes the heart and balances the mind

- Reduces stress; calms the nerves

- Neutralizes excessive heat and acidity in the stomach, colon, and liver

- Enhances absorption of nutrients

- Promotes a healthy glowing skin

- Supports healthy reproductive strength for both men and women

---

FENNEL MILK

Fennel Milk relieves hyperacidic or hot stomach excellently. It also calms the mind and nervous system, allowing you to fall asleep at night on time. Diluting whole milk with water makes it easier to digest without losing its valuable nutrients. Drink it alone in the morning or at night before going to bed.

½ cup spring water

½ cup whole milk

1 teaspoon fennel seeds

2 whole cloves

FOR AIRY DIGESTION: Add 2 crushed cardamom pods and a 1-inch piece of cinnamon stick.

FOR EARTHY DIGESTION: Add 2 crushed cardamom pods, a 1-inch piece of cinnamon stick, and 1 teaspoon grated fresh ginger.

Place all the ingredients in a small saucepan and bring to a boil over medium-high heat. Reduce the heat and simmer uncovered for 5 minutes. Strain and drink hot or warm.

NOTES

- If you have loose bowels, add ¼ teaspoon freshly grated nutmeg.

- **Dairy-free option:** Substitute almond milk (page 216) for the dairy milk.

- Fennel is estrogenic, so if you have concerns about estrogen, substitute coriander seeds for the fennel.

SUGGESTED COOLING MENUS

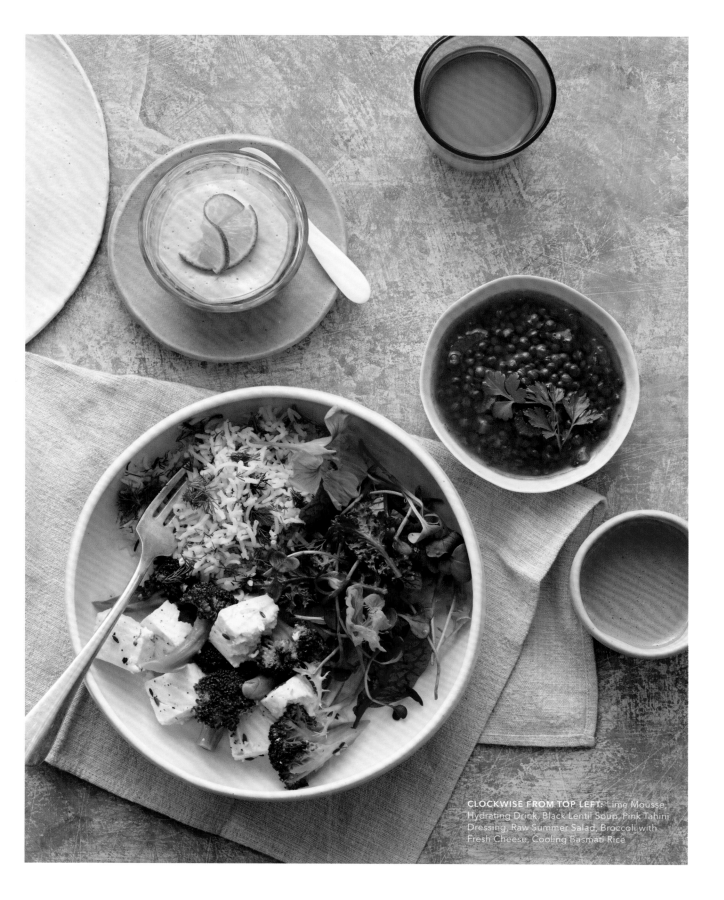

CLOCKWISE FROM TOP LEFT: Lime Mousse, Hydrating Drink, Black Lentil Soup, Pink Tahini Dressing, Raw Summer Salad, Broccoli with Fresh Cheese, Cooling Basmati Rice

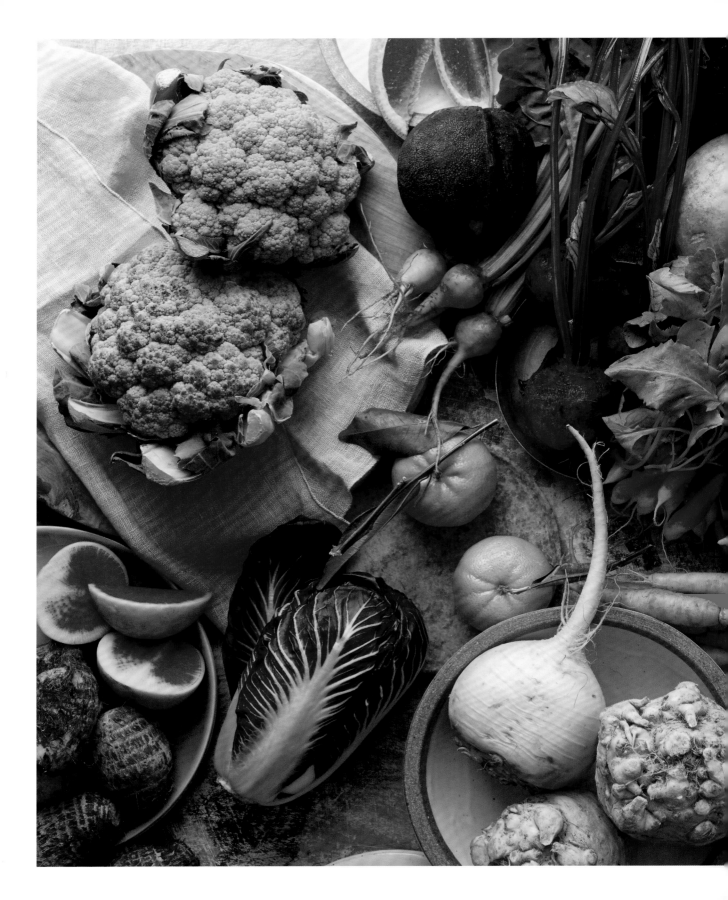

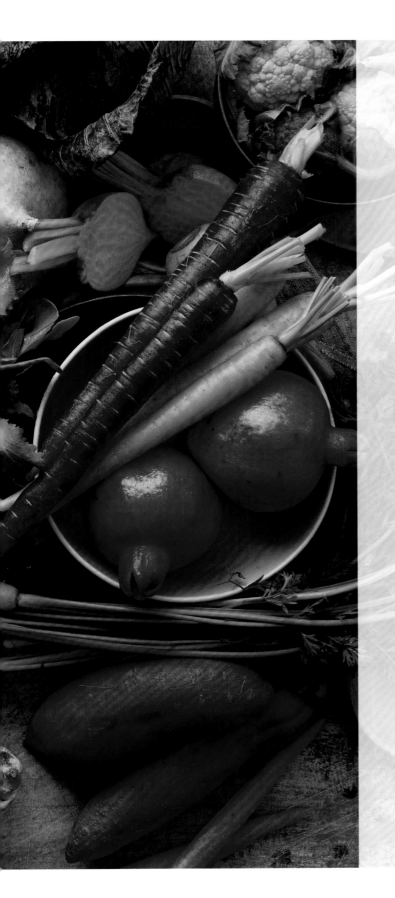

LATE FALL & WINTER

GROUNDING RECIPES

In late fall, when the temperatures drop below 65°F but are still above the freezing point, our systems continue to run on the heat energy accumulated during summer. As the weather chills and piercing cold winds take over and as our room heaters stay on, we will likely experience more dryness and lightness in our physiology. The cold temperature also shrinks our microcirculatory channels, which will slow down our circulation (causing those cold hands and feet) and increase the chances of blockages from undigested food residue.

To counter the cold in winter, our bodies have to work harder to produce more heat in order to maintain normal body temperature. During this time, fire in the stomach goes up, and that is why we need to fuel our bodies with foods that are heavier and richer in protein and fat. The challenge we may experience especially in late winter is that some heavier foods tend also to be clogging (such as winter squash, refined pastries, and other sweets), which could congest our already shrunken channels. If our circulation is poor, the increased digestive fire can get trapped in the stomach and not be properly distributed throughout the rest of the body. Trapped heat dries us from the inside, and cold winds dry us on the outside—this is one reason we tend to experience dry, flaky skin in winter. Following the recommendations below will help you stay balanced during the cold season until spring, when the daytime temperatures are between 45°F and 75°F.

Balance with vibrant, cooked foods that are heavy (good-quality dairy, basmati rice, einkorn, spelt), moist (soups, stews), oily (with ghee, olive oil), with warm, soft qualities and sweet, sour, and salty tastes (see "The Six Tastes of Food" on page 249) to appease your increased inner fire. You may also eat larger portions, but not more than you can digest easily. More food provides more heat for the body in cold weather. In this way your body will store good fats, proteins, and minerals so that you will have sustained energy to welcome nature's drastic changes in spring. Winter is "building season," and taking extra care of your health at this time will ensure overall good health for the rest of the year.

Stay away from foods of cold (raw, iced), light (popcorn, lettuce, puffed cereal), dry (crackers, yeasted bread, large beans) hard, rough qualities, carbonated drinks, and deep-fried food. Reduce foods of bitter, very pungent, and astringent tastes (see "The Six Tastes of Food" on page 249). Foods of predominantly bitter and astringent tastes may be too light and drying to feed the increased concentration of fire in the stomach and liver. Very pungent foods such as red chiles may burn and further accumulate heat and dryness in your digestive tract. Although foods of sweet taste balance us in winter, it doesn't mean you need to indulge in sweets. Eat sweets in moderation, as excessive sweetness can lower the digestive fire and lead to inflammation and weight gain. In this season, also avoid detoxing unless recommended by an expert and under close supervision. Cleansing in winter may aggravate and increase your digestive flame, which if not properly fed (as during fasting) will only burn your physiology more.

TIPS FOR IMPROVING AIRY DIGESTION

Revisit "Setting the Stage for Your Meals: It's Not Just What You Eat, But How You Eat It" on pages 40-41—this practice is always useful no matter what your digestion is. The following tips are specific for irregular Airy digestion:

- Follow the recipes and recommendations in this chapter.

- Chew 1 teaspoon After-Meal Spice Blend for Airy Digestion (at right) after lunch and dinner.

- Eat small meals at regular intervals (whenever you're hungry).

- Drink warm water throughout the day.

- Add extra ghee and olive oil to your food (avoid coconut oil because it's too cooling for this season).

- After a meal, rest for about 15 minutes and refrain from intensive physical activity.

- Do mild exercise daily for at least thirty minutes.

- Take a good-quality Triphala (Ayurvedic supplement) at night.

AFTER-MEAL SPICE BLEND FOR AIRY DIGESTION

This SV Ayurveda remedy has been passed down in the lineage for generations. Although fennel enhances digestive fire, its sweet, licorice-like taste balances the pungency of the spice so that it does not overheat the body. This makes it a helpful spice for when you're experiencing irregular Airy digestion.

Take this digestive aid every day and especially when you're traveling or eating out; it will give you almost immediate relief from bloating, colic pain, or gas. Chewing fennel seeds after every meal will also gradually improve your digestion. However, do not use this digestive aid as a quick fix for a poor diet. Good food is the foundation for good digestion, and fennel will support you along the way.

4 tablespoons fennel seeds

In a small heavy skillet, dry-toast 2 tablespoons of the fennel seeds over low heat until they darken a few shades and release their aroma; remove from the pan and let them cool down completely. Mix the toasted and raw fennel together and store in an airtight jar. Chew ½ teaspoon before and after every meal.

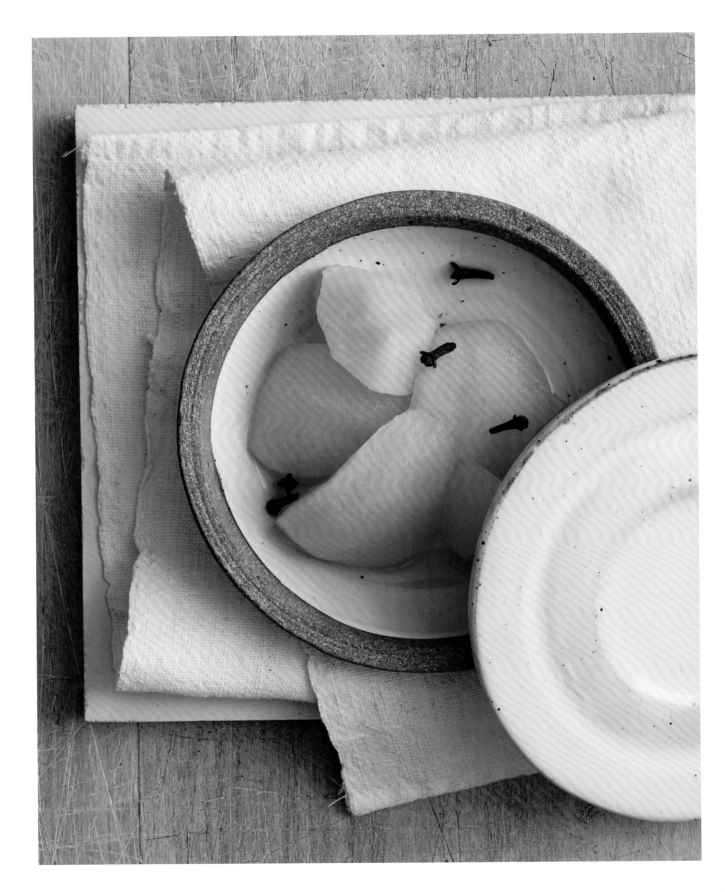

COOKED APPLE PRE-BREAKFAST

PREP: 1 MINUTE ■ **COOK:** 5 MINUTES   serves 1 `GF` `DF`

Single foods eaten at the right time can have the most profound effect on our health. When I first heard about Cooked Apple from Vaidya Mishra, I was skeptical—is it really so important to eat it first thing in the morning? Why cooked and not raw? After trying it a few times I loved it so much that to date, stewing an apple is part of my morning pre-breakfast ritual.

This is the easiest, fastest recipe in my book. Yet its benefits put to shame the most extravagant culinary creations in the world. I change my cooking class recipes seasonally, but I include Cooked Apple in every class handout. I am thrilled when students come back and tell me about their morning apple experience. So here is my challenge for you: if you are a beginner in the kitchen, start with this recipe—it will build your confidence. If you don't have time to cook, make this recipe anyway—it takes only a minute to prep and you can shower while it's cooking—it won't interfere with your rushed schedule. If you want to create lasting family memories for your kids, make them Cooked Apple—they will always remember waking up to the heavenly apple aroma.

Try this recipe and see how it works for you. Remember that the key is to eat it first thing in the morning, as close to the time you get up as possible.

2 whole cloves

1 medium apple, preferably a sweeter variety such as Golden Delicious, Gala, Fuji, Opal, or Pink Lady

FOR FIERY DIGESTION: Make as is or substitute a pear for the apple.

FOR EARTHY DIGESTION: Add a 1-inch piece cinnamon stick in Step 1.

1. Start boiling ½ cup water and the cloves in a small saucepan. In the meantime, peel, core, and chop the apple into bite-size pieces. If you don't have time to peel it, at least cut the apple into 4 pieces and remove the core.

2. Add the apple pieces to the hot water, bring to a boil, reduce the heat, cover, and simmer for 5 minutes, or until the apple is soft and translucent but not mushy.

3. Drain (you can reserve the liquid if you like—see Note), let it cool a little, and eat first thing in the morning.

NOTES

■ You may drink the cooking liquid as tea, add it to your oatmeal, or simply discard it.

■ Do not eat Cooked Apple if you have blood sugar issues.

SWEET POTATO SMOOTHIE

PREP: 1 MINUTE (WITH ALREADY MADE ALMOND MILK) ▪
COOK: 15 MINUTES

serves 1 or 2 (makes about 2 cups) GF DF

You might have doubts about whipping a sweet potato into a smoothie, but you will be thrilled to discover how delicious it is. Its delicate orange color, soft texture, and warming cozy effect will appease your airiness and ground you to your essence of bliss. Because it is filling but not heavy, I'll make this smoothie on a cold day for breakfast or at night when it is too late to eat a full meal but I still need to satisfy my hunger.

1 cup peeled and diced sweet potato or
jewel yam

½ teaspoon Sweet Masala (page 220)

6 strands saffron (optional)

1 or 2 Medjool dates or 2 to 3 smaller dates,
pitted and chopped

1 cup almond milk (page 216), plus more
if needed

¼ teaspoon vanilla extract

FOR FIERY DIGESTION: Omit the saffron and enjoy as is or substitute fresh coconut milk (page 217) for the almond milk.

FOR EARTHY DIGESTION: Omit the dates and add ¼ teaspoon ground cinnamon in Step 1.

1. Place the sweet potato, Sweet Masala, saffron, dates, and ½ cup water in a small saucepan. Bring to a boil, then reduce the heat to low, cover, and simmer for about 10 minutes, until the sweet potato is cooked through.

2. In a blender, combine the boiled sweet potato mixture, the almond milk, and vanilla and blend until very smooth. Add more water or almond milk to adjust to your preferred consistency.

3. Serve hot or warm.

NOTES

▪ If you don't have Sweet Masala handy, use a pinch each of ground cinnamon, cardamom, cloves, and nutmeg.

▪ For a more filling breakfast, add ¼ cup rolled oats plus ½ cup extra water in Step 1.

▪ You may substitute warm cow's milk for the almond milk.

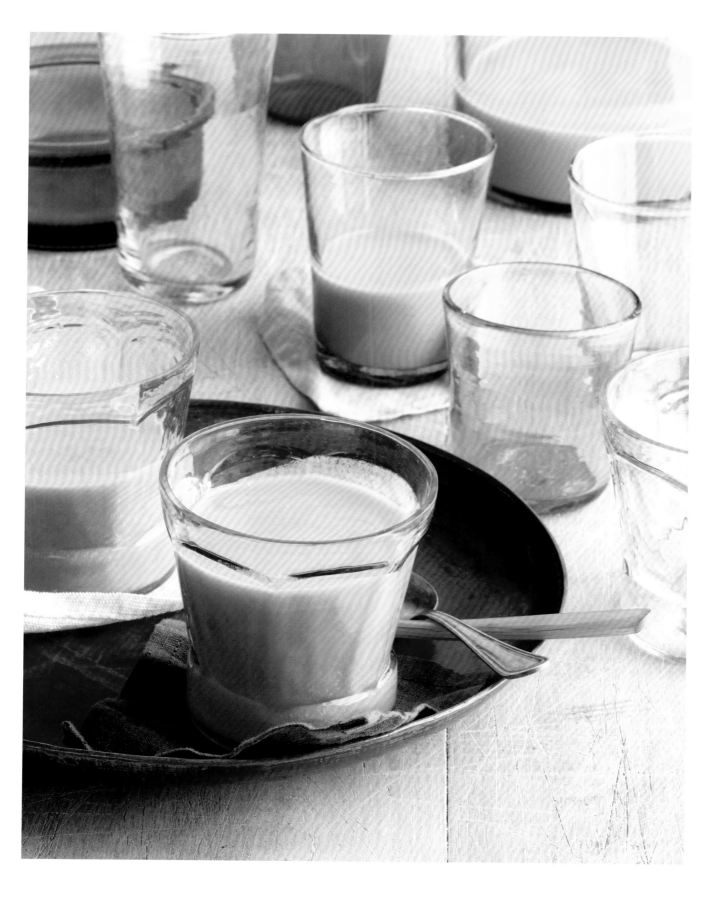

IRON SMOOTHIE

SOAK: AT LEAST 8 HOURS ▪ PREP: 5 TO 10 MINUTES   serves 1 or 2 (makes 2 to 3 cups) `GF` `DF`

I call this smoothie "iron" because its ingredients are rich in iron and other minerals, good fats, and protein. Its smooth texture feels silky in your mouth, leaving a pleasant aromatic aftertaste.

Dried fruits are suitable in winter through spring, when most fresh fruit is not in season. As they are dry and hard, dried fruit will make you more Airy; that's why it is important to soak and rehydrate them. So keep in mind that this is a recipe to start the night before—with soaking.

Enjoy this smoothie as an energy boost in the morning, afternoon, or when you expect a delay in eating a main meal.

3 dried apricots

3 dried black mission figs, stems removed

3 small pitted dates

3 pitted prunes

1 tablespoon raisins

10 raw almonds

2 tablespoons raw walnuts

2 cardamom pods, toasted

2 cups spring or filtered water

1 tablespoon fresh lime juice

> FOR FIERY DIGESTION: Add 1 teaspoon toasted, ground fennel seeds in Step 5.
>
> FOR EARTHY DIGESTION: Add a 1-inch piece of peeled and chopped ginger in Step 5. Do not use the water from soaking the dried fruit—it's too much sugar for you.

1. Place the dried fruit in a small bowl, cup, or jar, cover with boiling hot filtered water, and soak for at least 8 hours or overnight. Using boiling hot water is important to eliminate unfriendly microorganisms. Soak the almonds and walnuts in two separate containers with filtered room temperature water (best) or cold tap water. Keep everything refrigerated while soaking to prevent fermentation.

2. Drain the soaked dry fruit, reserving the liquid, and test it with your fingers to make sure there are no pieces of pits hiding in the prunes or dates; put the fruit in the blender. The soaking water captures a lot of the fruit's sugar—you can use it for blending or not, depending on how sweet you want your smoothie.

3. Strain and rinse the almonds and walnuts. Peel the almonds and add them to the blender along with the walnuts.

4. Add the cardamom, water, and lime juice and blend until smooth; if it's too thick, add more water to your preferred consistency. Slowly drink or eat with a spoon.

5. To store, transfer the smoothie to a jar or a bottle, cover, and refrigerate for up to 24 hours. For best digestion, enjoy it at room temperature.

NOTES

▪ For faster almond peeling, blanch the almonds in boiling hot water for seven seconds and drain immediately—this will keep the almonds raw, yet their skins will slip off easily.

▪ You may substitute one dried fruit for another if you do not have them all on hand.

AYURVEDIC TAKE ON OATMEAL

COOK: 12 TO 15 MINUTES

serves 1 GF DF

I meet a lot of people who religiously eat oatmeal for breakfast almost every day. The health benefits, easy preparation, and comforting nature of this inexpensive grain make it so appealing. I learned this recipe during my Ayurvedic training, and I play with its variations whenever I feel like eating good old oatmeal in the morning.

The cinnamon, cardamom, and saffron make bland oatmeal more enjoyable and help you digest the complex, slow-burning carbs and the proteins in the grain and milk, so you won't feel like you have a big lump in your stomach.

1 teaspoon ghee or coconut oil

2 cardamom pods, slightly crushed to open on one end

1-inch-long cinnamon stick

2 saffron threads (optional)

¼ cup rolled oats (see Notes)

½ cup water

½ cup cow's milk or almond milk (page 216)

1 Medjool date, pitted and finely chopped, or 1 tablespoon Thompson or golden raisins

FOR FIERY DIGESTION: Omit the saffron and substitute ¼ teaspoon ground fennel for the cinnamon stick.

FOR EARTHY DIGESTION: Oats might be too heavy for you, so you could replace them with barley flakes and cook them in ¾ cup water (no milk). If you want to stick with oats, omit the ghee and substitute water for the milk; add ¼ teaspoon powdered ginger with the water in Step 2.

1. In a small saucepan, heat the ghee over medium-low heat. Add the cardamom pods and cinnamon stick, and toast for about 1 minute, until the spices release their aroma and darken a shade. Add the saffron and oats, stir well, and toast for another 1 to 2 minutes, allowing the flakes to absorb the ghee.

2. Add the water, then the milk (adding the milk first might curdle it) and dates. Stir and bring to a full boil. Reduce the heat to low, partially cover, and cook for about 10 minutes, until the grains are cooked and creamy.

3. Turn off the heat and remove the cardamom pods and cinnamon stick. Serve hot.

NOTES

- To vary the seasonings, omit the cardamom and cinnamon and add Sweet Masala (page 220) in Step 2.

- To make your oatmeal with steel-cut oats, add at least ¼ cup more water in Step 2. This heartier style of oats will take 10 to 15 minutes longer to cook. You may also soak steel-cut oats overnight and drain them before cooking, which will make them lighter and speed up cooking time.

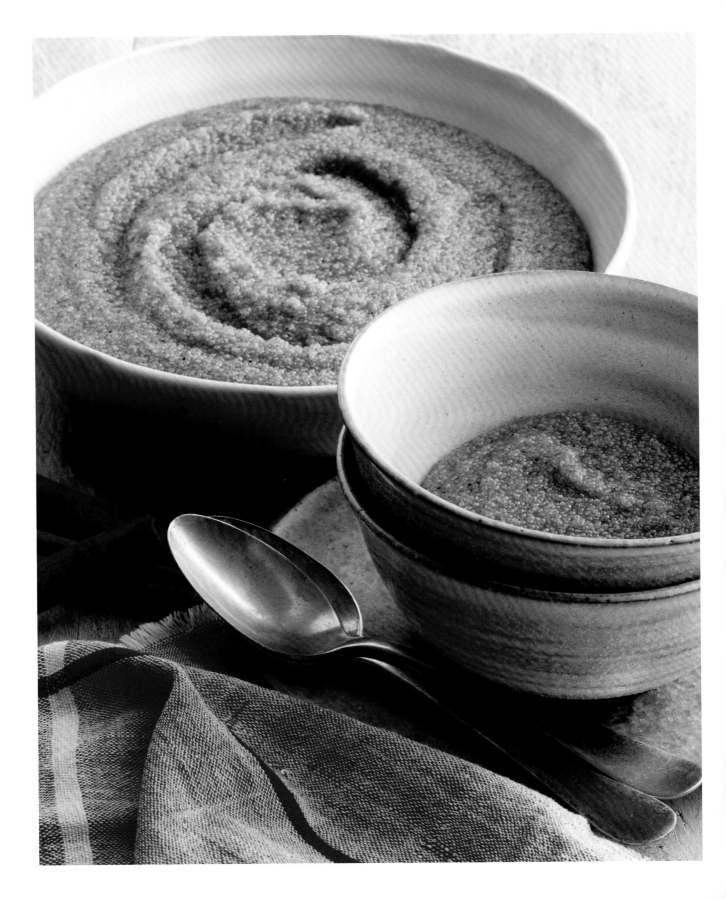

SPICED AMARANTH

COOK: 20 TO 25 MINUTES

What is your relationship with amaranth? Are you like I was a few years ago—you completely ignore it on the grocery shelves? Until I discovered how much I loved amaranth, I passed it by, like passing by a celebrity neighbor until you realize, "Ah, that's you!"

This tiny grain definitely makes the grade as a celebrity among foods, and even though it has been cooked in civilizations throughout the world for more than eight thousand years, it seems to be served less often on American tables. Well, be brave and try this recipe because amaranth is delicious and its nutrients are just too important to ignore.

Because it is one of the most protein-rich plant-based foods, amaranth can be harder for some people to digest. The spices I use in this recipe not only complement amaranth's earthy, nutty flavor, but also aid digestion. The key to a successful amaranth dish is to cook it just enough, to a creamy-sticky consistency. Overcooking it will make it hard to chew. If you've ever eaten the Indian dessert called halava (semolina pudding), you can aim for your cooked amaranth to look like a creamy halava. Let your eyes be smaller than your stomach and serve smaller portions—amaranth is much denser than most grains, and just a little will satiate you. You can serve this dish as a breakfast cereal or as a grain dish to accompany any vegetable dish or salad.

½ teaspoon kalonji seeds

¼ teaspoon ajwain seeds

¼ teaspoon black peppercorns

1 cup amaranth (no need to wash)

1-inch piece cinnamon stick

½ teaspoon salt

2 teaspoons ghee or olive oil

Sprinkle of lime juice

FOR FIERY DIGESTION: Substitute coconut oil for the ghee; omit the ajwain seeds and add 1 teaspoon fennel or coriander seeds in Step 1.

FOR EARTHY DIGESTION: Add 1 teaspoon grated fresh ginger in Step 2. Omit the olive oil in Step 3.

1. In a spice grinder, grind the kalonji seeds, ajwain seeds, and black peppercorns to a fine powder.

2. In a 1- to 2-quart saucepan, combine 2 cups water, amaranth, cinnamon stick, salt, ghee, and ground spices to a boil. Reduce the heat to low, cover with a tight-fitting lid, and simmer for 20 to 25 minutes, until the grains have thickened to a creamy consistency. I like to keep an eye on the consistency

by giving the bubbly amaranth a quick stir every 10 minutes. Once you've reached 20 minutes cooking time, you will see a little bit of water on the surface, but as soon as you stir the grains, they will absorb the water and you will achieve the perfect creamy, slightly sticky grain texture.

3. Turn off the heat leaving the pot covered, and let the grains firm up for 5 more minutes. Garnish with a squeeze of lime juice; serve hot.

VARIATION

- Substitute ¼ cup red or white quinoa (wash it well) for ¼ cup of the amaranth in Step 2.

The Healing Benefits of Amaranth

The Greeks called it "immortal," and the Aztecs revered it as "golden grain of the gods." These are some of amaranth's benefits (they refer to the amaranth grain—technically a seed—the amaranth greens are also delicious but have different nutrient ratios and healing properties).

- It is a source of complete protein—it contains all the essential amino acids, including lysine, which is lacking in most grains.

- It is high in fiber and a good source of magnesium and iron.

- It is rich in manganese, calcium, magnesium, phosphorus, and potassium.

- It is an ideal grain for vegetarians, vegans, and diabetics.

SCRAMBLED CHEESE

PREP: 5 MINUTES ▪ **COOK:** ABOUT 10 MINUTES
(WITH ALREADY MADE CHEESE AND MASALA)

serves 3 to 4 **GF**

Every time we make it in class, my students exclaim, "It looks like scrambled eggs!" The heaviness of the cheese resembles the texture of eggs, and the sulfury black salt gives this dish the eggy flavor. The rest of the seasonings enhance deliciousness and support digestion of cheese.

Serve Scrambled Cheese with a non-starchy salad, cooked greens, a light grain, and a dab of Raisin-Cranberry Sauce (page 189), Daikon Radish Chutney (page 192), or Cilantro Chutney (page 191).

2 cups very soft fresh cheese
 (page 202), strained for 15 minutes
 and crumbled

1 tablespoon ghee

½ teaspoon ground turmeric

½ teaspoon cumin seeds

⅛ teaspoon asafoetida

1 teaspoon Digestive Masala (page 223)

½ teaspoon black salt

¼ teaspoon salt

1 cup grated zucchini or thinly sliced celery

¼ teaspoon coarsely ground black pepper

1 tablespoon chopped fresh parsley leaves

1 teaspoon minced fresh rosemary, or 2 small
 pinches dried rosemary

FOR FIERY DIGESTION: Omit the black salt and asafoetida; substitute Cooling Masala (page 221) for the Digestive Masala; add more zucchini if you like.

FOR EARTHY DIGESTION: Reduce the ghee to 1 teaspoon; substitute Energizing Masala (page 221) for the Digestive Masala; add a minced green Thai chile with the asafoetida in Step 2; add more rosemary in Step 3; enjoy a smaller portion.

1. Place ⅓ cup of the crumbled cheese in a blender, add ¼ to ⅓ cup water, and blend into a smooth sauce that resembles heavy cream.

2. In a pan, heat the ghee over low heat. Add the turmeric and toast for 15 seconds, then add the cumin seeds and toast until they release their aroma. Add the asafoetida, masala, and both salts, followed immediately by the zucchini. Sauté for 2 to 3 minutes (do not cover). Stir in the crumbled cheese and the blended cheese cream and cook, stirring occasionally, for 5 minutes, or until everything is well incorporated with a creamy-lumpy texture. Turn off the heat.

3. Fold in the pepper, parsley, and rosemary. Serve immediately.

NOTE

▪ I always feel like sprinkling a pinch of paprika over this dish, but alas, paprika, made from dried red peppers, is a nightshade concentrate! Well, occasionally I'll break the SV Ayurveda rules and use it. A handful of baby arugula folded in in Step 3 is quite nice.

TURMERIC RICE

PREP: 10 MINUTES ■ **COOK:** 20 MINUTES   serves 4 **GF** **DF**

It was during my initial visit to a yoga studio in my hometown of Plovdiv, Bulgaria, that I first marveled at the bright yellow color of cooked rice. At that time there were no Indian restaurants around, and turmeric was foreign to Bulgarian cooking. Today turmeric is easily available in grocery stores all over the world. It not only colors food yellow, but also adds an earthy flavor to dishes, especially rice. Go to page 231 to learn more about the incredible benefits of turmeric.

Make Turmeric Rice shine as a supporting companion to Red Velvet Soup (page 162), Kale and Roasted Sweet Potatoes (page 173), or Sautéed Leafy Greens (page 118).

1 cup white basmati rice

1 teaspoon salt

½ teaspoon ground turmeric

4 whole cloves

3 teaspoons ghee or coconut oil

6 curry leaves

> **FOR FIERY DIGESTION:** Reduce the turmeric to ¼ teaspoon.
>
> **FOR EARTHY DIGESTION:** Omit the ghee and add a ½-inch cinnamon stick in Step 2; reduce the ghee to 1 teaspoon in Step 4.

1. Using a mesh strainer, rinse the rice and soak it in cold water for 10 minutes; drain well.

2. In a 1- to 2-quart saucepan, bring 2 cups water to a boil and add the salt, turmeric, cloves, and 1 teaspoon of the ghee. Add the rice and return to a full boil.

3. Cover with a tight-fitting lid, reduce the heat to low, and simmer for 15 minutes. Do not open or stir the pot. In 15 minutes, check whether the grains need a little more water or more time—all the water should be absorbed, and a grain of rice should not be hard when squeezed between your two fingers. Turn off the heat and keep the grains covered.

4. In a metal measuring cup or a small pan, heat the remaining 2 teaspoons ghee over medium-low heat, add the curry leaves, and sauté for 5 to 10 seconds, until the leaves crisp up. Drizzle the infused ghee and leaves on the rice, cover, and let the grains firm up for 5 more minutes.

5. Fluff with a fork and remove the cloves and curry leaves. Serve steamy hot.

NOTE

■ Here's an alternative method of cooking that adds a nuance of toasted flavor and more warming energy to the rice: Pat-dry the washed and soaked rice in Step 1. Heat 1 tablespoon ghee over low heat, add the turmeric, cloves, and curry leaves, and cook for 10 to 15 seconds. Add the rice and gently stir-fry until the grains become translucent and squeaky. Add the water and salt and follow the cooking instructions in Step 3. Skip Step 4.

Turmeric Facial Mask

Beyond gorgeous glow, this mask makes your skin feel luxurious to the touch. It even helps to remove unwanted facial hairs and peach fuzz, for the ultimate skin-smoothing effect. This recipe makes enough to cover the face, neck, and décolletage. It is best to use the mask as soon as you make it because it thickens as it sits.

½ teaspoon ground turmeric

2 teaspoons chickpea flour (for sensitive-oily skin) or oat flour (for dry or combination skin)

2 teaspoons sweet almond oil or olive oil

1 teaspoon raw milk, almond milk (page 216), or rose water

1. Mix the ingredients in a bowl or a blender until they form a thick paste.

2. Apply a thick layer of the mask directly to your face, neck, and décolletage.

3. Let dry for 15 to 20 minutes, until the mask begins to crack.

4. Rinse off with warm water and a wash-cloth. Look in the mirror and marvel.

HOW THE INGREDIENTS ACT

- Turmeric is an anti-inflammatory agent that removes redness, reduces puffiness, and even stimulates circulation (meaning it also helps to boost collagen production for a more youthful appearance).

- Chickpea flour absorbs excess oil (so you look luminous, not shiny) and serves to exfoliate the skin's surface.

- Oat flour boosts hydration and brings softness to dry skin.

- Sweet almond oil and olive oil moisturize deep down, smoothing out lines and wrinkles and giving the skin a lustrous, dewy glow.

- Raw milk, almond milk, and rose water soften, hydrate, and give the skin a boost of radiance.

Grandma's Turmeric Stain Remover

Turmeric stains are hard to get rid of, even with dry cleaning. Here is the old Indian grandma's remedy: do not wet or wash the stained garment. Expose it to direct sunlight for a few hours—the stain will magically disappear!

STIR-FRIED RED AND BLACK RICE

SOAK: 30 MINUTES ▪ **PREP:** 5 MINUTES ▪ **COOK:** ABOUT 40 MINUTES   serves 4

David Frenkiel and Luise Vindahl inspired me to "Ayurvedize" their recipe for Stir-Fried Red Rice (published in *Green Kitchen Travels*). I really enjoy reading their books and their family cooking blog, www.GreenKitchenStories.com.

The Ayurvedic texts glorify red rice as one of the best types of rice because it is low glycemic and balancing for everybody. It is the only whole-grain rice that cooks in twenty minutes! Black rice (aka forbidden rice) originated in ancient China, where it was known as "longevity rice" and was reserved for the emperors. Both varieties are an excellent source of minerals including manganese, magnesium, potassium, molybdenum, and phosphorus.

Stir-Fried Red and Black Rice looks like a piece of art, a hand-woven carpet, a true feast for the eyes and taste buds. The deep purple black rice stands out against the background of the russet-colored red rice, highlighted with patches of green, orange, and white from the vegetables and nuts. Add to this picture the roasted nutty rice flavor enhanced by seasonings and your senses will be completely satisfied.

This recipe demonstrates how you can apply Ayurvedic principles to Asian-style cooking. Accompanied by Cilantro Chutney (page 191) or Sunflower-Sesame Dip (page 197), it makes a satisfying meal on its own, but it also goes well with Sautéed Leafy Greens (page 118) or Broccoli Rabe and Cauliflower (page 70).

¼ cup black rice, rinsed, soaked for 30 minutes, and drained

¾ cup Bhutanese red rice, rinsed, soaked for 30 minutes, and drained

1½ teaspoons salt

1 tablespoon ghee, sesame oil, or coconut oil

1 tablespoon thinly julienned fresh ginger

1 teaspoon ground coriander

Small pinch of asafoetida

1 medium-large carrot, cut into ¼-inch-wide, 2-inch-long strips (about 1 cup)

2 celery sticks or fennel stalks, thinly sliced (about 1 cup)

1 head baby bok choy or ¼ Chinese cabbage, sliced ½-inch thick (about 2 cups)

¼ teaspoon freshly ground black pepper

GARNISHES

1 teaspoon ghee, sesame oil, or coconut oil

⅓ cup raw cashews

Small handful fresh basil leaves, torn into pieces (optional)

FOR FIERY DIGESTION: Omit the fresh ginger or replace it with 1 teaspoon powdered sunthi ginger (see page 89).

FOR EARTHY DIGESTION: Use sesame oil for cooking. Add 1 or 2 green Thai chiles, cut into thin strips, with the ginger in Step 3. Omit the toasted nuts in Step 4.

(CONTINUED)

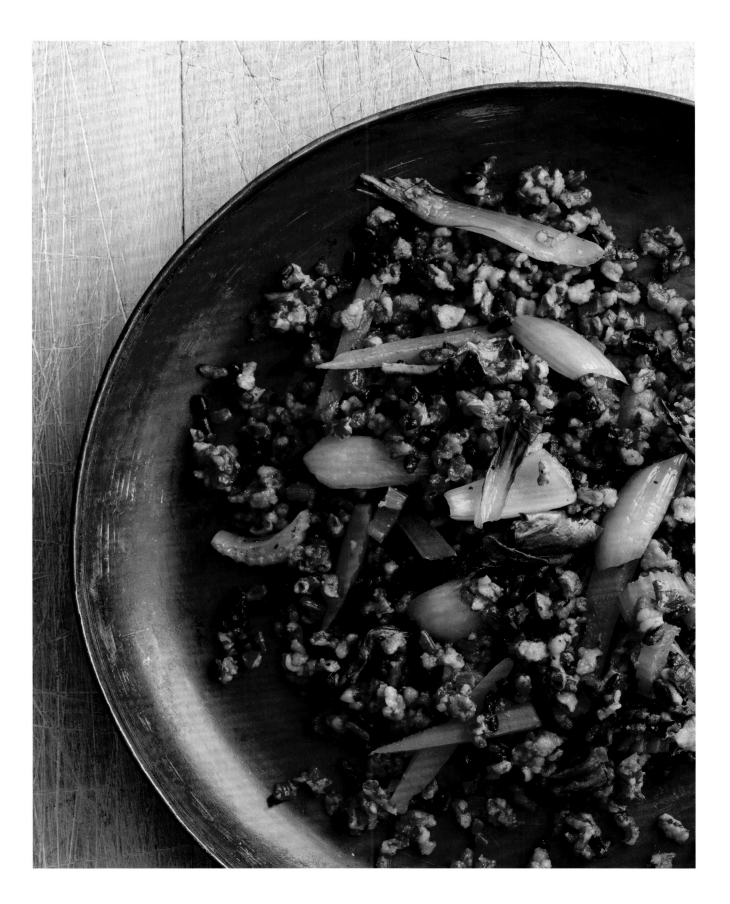

1. Combine the black rice with 1½ cups water and ¼ teaspoon salt. Bring to a boil over medium-high heat, then lower the heat, cover, and simmer for 30 to 40 minutes, until the grains are soft. Drain any excess water and set aside uncovered for 5 minutes to let the grains firm up. Fluff with a fork.

2. In another small saucepan, combine the red rice with 2 cups water and ¾ of the teaspoon salt. Bring to a simmer over medium-high heat, then lower the heat, cover, and simmer for 20 minutes, or until the grains are soft. Drain any excess water and set aside uncovered for 5 minutes to let the grains firm up. Fluff with a fork.

3. While the rice is cooking, heat the 1 tablespoon ghee in a wok or skillet over high heat. Add the ginger and crisp it for 15 seconds, then add the following ingredients in consecutive order: the coriander, asafoetida, ½ teaspoon salt, carrot, celery, and bok choy. Stir-fry for 5 to 10 minutes, until the vegetables are crisp-tender and slightly browned in parts. You may cover the pan with a lid for the last 3 minutes to speed up the cooking. Season with the pepper. Add the cooked black rice and red rice, reduce the heat to medium-high, and stir-fry for another 3 to 4 minutes, until the grains are warmed through.

4. In a small skillet, heat the 1 teaspoon ghee over medium heat. Add the cashews and toast until they turn lightly golden, 3 to 4 minutes.

5. Garnish the dish with the cashews and basil leaves and serve hot.

NOTE

- I choose to cook the black and the red rice separately in order to preserve their distinct colors. If you cook the two together, the black rice will overpower the red rice with its deep purple color.

VARIATIONS

- Substitute ¼ cup additional red rice for the black rice and cook it together with the remaining red rice, increasing the water to 2¼ cups and the salt to 1 teaspoon in Step 2 (skip Step 1).

- Substitute chopped spinach for the bok choy— add it in the last 2 minutes of stir-frying the vegetables.

GROUNDING KHICHARI (RICE AND LENTIL STEW)

SOAK: 30 MINUTES ▪ **PREP:** 10 MINUTES ▪ **COOK:** 40 MINUTES   serves 4 `GF` `DF`

Here is my grounding and warming version of this meal-in-a-pot dish. You can easily prepare it in a slow cooker by starting it at night on low, then in the morning pack the ready khichari in a thermos and take it to work. Grounding Khichari goes well with any of the chutneys on pages 191 to 192, with steamed salads, and with cooked leafy greens.

½ cup yellow split mung dal or red lentils

1 cup basmati rice

1 tablespoon ghee, sesame oil, or olive oil

½ teaspoon ground turmeric

1 tablespoon grated fresh ginger

6 curry leaves or 2 bay leaves

1 small green Thai chile, seeded and minced

2½ teaspoons Grounding Masala (page 222)

2 teaspoons salt

2 cups diced vegetables (you can combine a few), such as carrots, sweet potatoes, taro root, green beans, zucchini, celery root, beets, and/or leafy greens

GARNISHES

1 tablespoon olive oil

Cracked black pepper

3 tablespoons chopped fresh cilantro, basil, dill, or parsley

Lime slices

FOR FIERY DIGESTION: Substitute Cooling Masala (page 221) or Superspice Masala (page 219) for the Grounding Masala; omit the ginger and chile in Step 2.

FOR EARTHY DIGESTION: Substitute quinoa for the rice in Step 1. Substitute Energizing Masala (page 221) for the Grounding Masala; add one more chile in Step 2. Omit the olive oil in Step 3.

1. Soak the dal and rice in a bowl together for 30 minutes. Rinse until the water runs clear and drain well.

2. Heat the ghee in a heavy 4-quart saucepan over low heat. Add the turmeric and toast for 10 seconds, then add the ginger, curry leaves, and chile and continue to toast until they crisp up, about 30 seconds. Add the rice and dal and stir frequently until the dal is almost dry. Add the masala, salt, vegetables, and 4 to 5 cups water. (Add quick-cooking vegetables such as zucchini, asparagus, or leafy greens 30 minutes into the cooking.) Bring to a full boil, then cover, reduce the heat to low, and simmer, stirring occasionally, for about 40 minutes, until the lentils begin to dissolve, the rice is soft, and the vegetables are cooked. If the khichari dries out too much and begins to stick to the bottom of the pot, add more water; you're looking for a creamy, moist consistency.

3. Garnish the khichari with olive oil, a few turns of cracked pepper, and the cilantro. Serve hot with lime slices alongside.

VARIATION

▪ For deeper cleansing, substitute ¼ cup soaked and ground (to a paste) kulthi beans (page 69, Step 1) for ¼ cup of the yellow split mung dal.

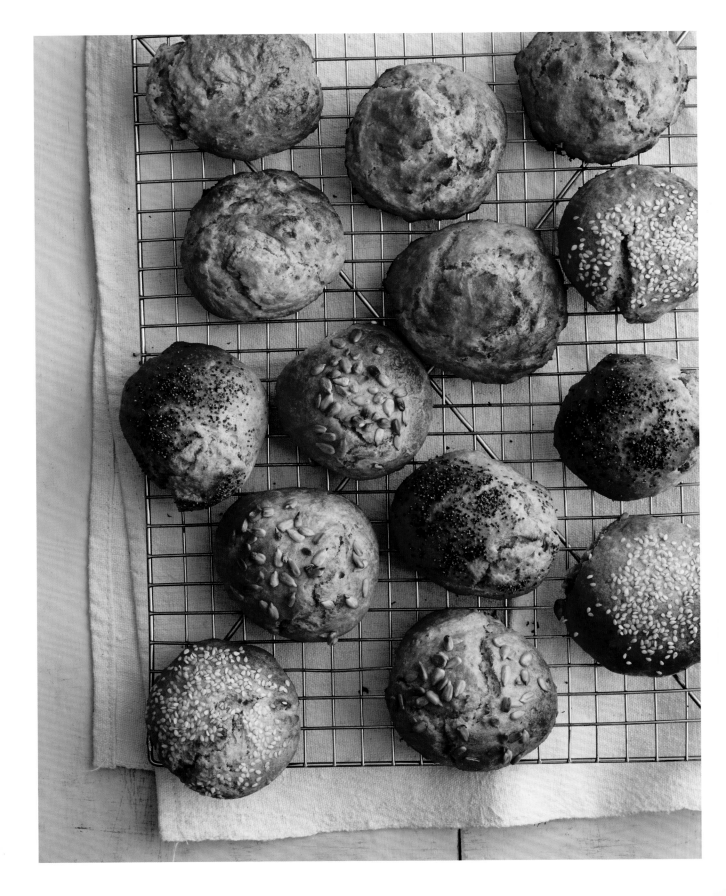

EINKORN BARLEY BISCUITS

PREP: 5 MINUTES ▪ **BAKE:** 10 TO 25 MINUTES, DEPENDING ON THE TEMPERATURE YOU CHOOSE

makes 6 large or 9 small biscuits **GF** **DF**

I was twenty-one and a novice cook at the yoga ashram in Bulgaria when something life-changing happened: my spiritual mentor, Krishna Kshetra Swami (aka Dr. Kenneth Valpey), came to visit. It was the first time I cooked for him, and I was so nervous. At the end of his visit, he gave me cooking advice that I still follow and share with you in this book.

In my sincere efforts to cook healthy food for my teacher, I made eggless, whole wheat, yeast-free biscuits—apparently they turned so hard that when he took one and knocked it on the table, it sounded like rock! Nevertheless, he kept smiling and compassionately accepted everything I made for him. On that day, I decided to learn to become an expert chef in service to others. It was the stone-hard biscuits that hammered this determination into my heart and transformed me into a life-long learner in the kitchen.

Twenty-five years later, I have my upgraded biscuit recipe to share with you. With just a few simple ingredients you can quickly create wholesome, soft, and tasty little breads that go well with soups and non-starchy vegetables.

1½ cups (184 grams) whole einkorn flour

¾ cup (91 grams) barley flour

1½ teaspoons baking powder

½ teaspoon salt

¼ teaspoon baking soda

1 cup buttermilk or water, plus 2 tablespoons buttermilk for brushing

¼ cup melted ghee or olive oil

1 tablespoon fresh lime juice

FOR FIERY DIGESTION: Enjoy them as they are.

FOR EARTHY DIGESTION: Substitute rye flour (225 grams) for the einkorn flour; add an additional 2 to 3 tablespoons buttermilk or water in Step 3. Enjoy smaller portions, occasionally.

1. Preheat the oven to 425°F if using ghee or 350°F if using olive oil. Grease a baking sheet.

2. In a medium bowl, sift or whisk together the flours, baking powder, salt, and baking soda.

3. In a separate bowl, whisk together the buttermilk, ghee, and lime juice.

4. Add the wet ingredients to the dry ingredients and lightly stir with a few strokes, just enough to make a smooth dough (overmixing will make your biscuits stiff).

5. Wet your hands and gently shape the dough into six larger bread rolls or nine smaller ones and line them up on the baking sheet. Feel free to play with the shape. For a golden crust, brush them with buttermilk.

6. Bake for 8 to 10 minutes at 425°F or 20 to 25 minutes at 350°F, until slightly crusty and golden on top and bottom. Cool the biscuits on a wire rack. Serve warm or at room temperature.

(CONTINUED)

NOTES

- Einkorn flour is sold in some health food stores and it is easily available online. Jovial Foods and Tropical Traditions are good brands.

- Sifting the dry ingredients helps to evenly mix in the leaveners, which results in softer, airy biscuits. Another way of sifting is to spin the dry ingredients in a food processor or a standing mixer or with a hand mixer for 5 to 10 seconds.

- To make a loaf of bread, multiply the recipe by one and a half and bake in a well-greased 1½-pound loaf pan in a preheated 350°F oven for about 40 minutes, until the bread has a golden crust and a skewer inserted in the middle of the loaf comes out clean.

FLOUR VARIATIONS

- **Only einkorn flour:** Use 2½ cups (300 grams) whole-grain einkorn flour.

- Substitute whole spelt or whole wheat flour for the einkorn flour. Add ¼ cup extra buttermilk or water for a soft, sticky dough, wet enough to shape into biscuits.

- **Gluten-free option:** Substitute 1½ cups (225 grams) buckwheat flour for the einkorn and barley flours.

FLAVORINGS (ADD IN STEP 1)

- 1 teaspoon dried herbs such as basil, thyme, Italian seasoning, rosemary, and/or savory

- 1 teaspoon caraway, kalonji, ajwain, or blue poppy seeds

- ¼ cup sunflower seeds or sesame seeds

To decorate, brush the biscuits with buttermilk and sprinkle a few pinches of the flavoring you chose for the dough on top.

Einkorn, the Ancestor Wheat

Throughout the history of agriculture, wheat has been cultivated and hybridized to increase yield, pest resistance, and elasticity in baked goods. As a result, today's wheat has a much more complex genetic makeup, which makes it very hard to digest. To challenge our digestion even more, most of the nonorganic wheat in the United States is "Roundup Ready," which means its genes have been altered to withstand the patented weed killer Roundup, a potent herbicide. The more the genetic structure of the grain has been manipulated, the more likely that its proteins can cause intestinal distress. No wonder we have such an explosion of gluten intolerance!

Einkorn was one of the first foods planted, at the dawn of agriculture ten thousand years ago, and the genetics of einkorn wheat haven't changed since these ancient times. It is considered a pure form of wheat that is more nutritious and tastes and digests in the body the way nature intended. In English, we borrow the word *einkorn* from the German, meaning "single grain"; that's because einkorn only has one grain attached to the stem, while other wheat varieties have groups of four grains.

Einkorn is incredibly delicious and easy to cook with, though some adjustments may be needed when converting recipes from contemporary wheat to einkorn. Bread dough made with einkorn can be very sticky, while cake batters sometimes can get gummy with mixing. Visit www.jovialfoods.com for useful baking tips and more einkorn recipes.

WINTER VEGETABLE STOCK

PREP: 5 MINUTES ▪ **COOK:** 40 MINUTES   makes about 4 cups `GF` `DF`

Extracting the flavor of vegetables and herbs to create an aromatic base for soups, sauces, and other preparations has been practiced in kitchens for hundreds of years. Today we tend to replace homemade stock with the more convenient premade bouillon, but I find that the exuberant flavor of freshly simmered vegetables is motivating enough to tune me back into the good old practice of stock making. Although most stocks are simmered uncovered to allow evaporation and concentration, I choose to cook this stock covered because my goal is different: to keep the liquid volume intact and lock in the flavors.

I use this stock to round up the seasoning for Braised Root Vegetables (page 167), and you can substitute an equal amount of it for any of the soups in this chapter. Winter Vegetable Stock is also an excellent nourishing broth for when you're feeling congested or feverish and don't feel like eating or when you're recovering from surgery.

2 teaspoons ghee or olive oil

1 tablespoon grated fresh ginger

1-inch cinnamon stick

10 black peppercorns

½ teaspoon cumin seeds

1 teaspoon salt

1 celery stalk, thinly sliced

1 cup thinly sliced fennel stalk, fennel bulb, or broccoli stems

2 small taro roots or 1 medium parsnip, peeled and diced

10 sprigs fresh cilantro

4 sprigs fresh basil

FOR FIERY DIGESTION: Omit the ginger; add 1 teaspoon fennel seeds and 1 teaspoon coriander seeds as you toast the spices in Step 1.

FOR EARTHY DIGESTION: Add 1 minced green Thai chile as you toast the spices in Step 1.

1. Heat the ghee in a 3- to 4-quart saucepan over medium-low heat. Add the ginger, cinnamon, peppercorns, and cumin and toast for 10 to 15 seconds, until the spices release their aroma. Add salt, celery, fennel, and taro and sauté, stirring occasionally, for 4 to 5 minutes—this step adds new flavor and activates the fat-soluble aromatic molecules of the ingredients.

2. Add 4 cups water, cilantro, and basil, cover, and bring to a full boil. Reduce the heat and simmer for 30 minutes. Strain and discard the vegetables, reserving the stock.

3. To store, keep refrigerated in a covered container for up to 48 hours.

RED VELVET SOUP

SOAK: 30 MINUTES ▪ **PREP:** 5 MINUTES ▪ **COOK:** 30 MINUTES   serves 4 GF DF

If you've been on the Airy side for a long time, you may not only have the typical cold hands and feet, but you may occasionally feel drained and even be anemic. Stressful schedules and cold weather can do that to us, so I created this protein- and iron-rich soup to boost our strength and add a little extra redness to our cheeks. It is also suitable to include in your diet when recovering from surgery, illness, or childbirth.

   With its bold color and potent yet gentle seasoning, Red Velvet Soup makes quite a statement. It will warm you up and brighten your table on a cold and gloomy day.

2 teaspoons coriander seeds

½ teaspoon cumin seeds

1 cup red lentils, washed, soaked for 30 minutes, drained, and rinsed

2 medium red beets, peeled and cut into 1-inch cubes (about 2½ cups)

½ teaspoon ground turmeric

1 large or 2 small bay leaves or cassia leaves

1 small green Thai chile, seeded and minced

1 tablespoon ghee or olive oil

2 teaspoons salt

1 tablespoon olive oil

¼ teaspoon freshly ground black pepper

GARNISHES

1 tablespoon coarsely chopped fresh cilantro leaves

½ teaspoon Cooling Pungent Masala (page 222), or to taste

4 lime slices

> **FOR FIERY DIGESTION:** Reduce the turmeric to ¼ teaspoon, substitute 6 curry leaves for the bay leaves, omit the chile and black pepper, and garnish with extra cilantro.
>
> **FOR EARTHY DIGESTION:** Reduce the ghee and olive oil to 1 teaspoon each; add ¼ teaspoon asafoetida and one more green Thai chile with the other spices in Step 2.

1. Grind the coriander and cumin seeds to a fine powder in a spice grinder.

2. Combine the red lentils and 4 cups water in a heavy 3-quart saucepan. Bring to a full boil over high heat, stirring occasionally. Remove any froth from the surface (this will reduce the gassiness of the lentils). Add the ground coriander and cumin, the beets, turmeric, bay leaves, chile, and ghee and mix well. Bring to a boil again, then reduce the heat to medium-low, cover with a tight-fitting lid, and simmer until the lentils and beets are soft and cooked through, about 20 minutes.

3. Turn off the heat and leave the pot uncovered to allow the soup to cool down a bit. Remove the bay leaves and add the salt, olive oil, and black pepper. Blend the soup to a more chunky or smooth consistency; you may also add more water if you like—in this case, adjust the salt to taste.

4. Garnish with the cilantro and Cooling Pungent Masala, and serve hot with lime slices. The lime enhances the taste and helps with protein digestion and iron absorption.

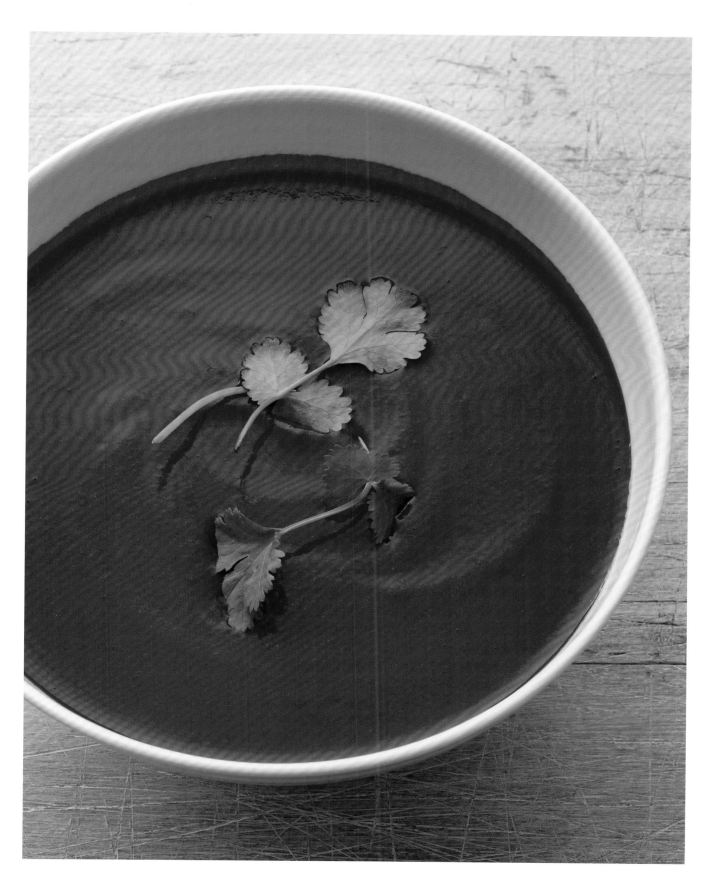

SOOTHING MUNG SOUP

SOAK: 30 MINUTES ▪ **COOK:** 30 TO 40 MINUTES

serves 4 `GF` `DF`

The number of *hmmms* and *yums* we hear every time we serve this traditional Ayurvedic soup (aka dal) in our classes or at events always amuses me. There is something about its smoothness, lightness, accent flavors, and bright yellow color! This recipe is easy on all levels—from gathering the ingredients, to preparation, to digestion. Make this soup to calm down and "land" after traveling or at the end of a long, stressful day. It goes well with rice, vegetables, and chutney.

1 cup yellow split mung dal

2 tablespoons ghee or sesame oil

½ teaspoon ground turmeric

6 curry leaves or 2 bay or cassia leaves

1½ teaspoons peeled, finely grated or minced fresh ginger

2 teaspoons ground coriander

1¼ teaspoons salt

GARNISHES

½ teaspoon cumin seeds

1 tablespoon olive oil

2 tablespoons coarsely chopped fresh cilantro or minced fresh dill

A few turns of the pepper mill

4 lime slices

FOR FIERY DIGESTION: Reduce the turmeric to ¼ teaspoon and omit the ginger in Step 2; garnish with extra cilantro.

FOR EARTHY DIGESTION: Substitute sesame oil for the ghee or reduce the ghee to 1 teaspoon in Step 2 and Step 5. Add 1 or 2 seeded and minced green Thai chiles with the ginger in Step 2.

1. Soak the mung dal for 30 minutes, then drain and rinse well.

2. Heat 1 tablespoon of the ghee in a heavy 2-quart saucepan over low heat. Add the turmeric and toast for 10 seconds, then add the curry leaves and ginger and continue to toast until they crisp up, about 30 seconds. Add the coriander and mung dal, then stir frequently until the lentils are almost dry (cooking the lentils this way reduces their lectin levels).

3. Add 4 cups water and bring the soup to a full boil, then cover, reduce the heat, and simmer, stirring occasionally, for 30 minutes, or until the mung dal begins to disintegrate.

4. Turn off the heat, add the salt, and beat with a wire whisk until the soup is creamy smooth. You may add more water if you like a lighter consistency; if you do, adjust the salt to taste.

5. Heat the remaining 1 tablespoon ghee in a small pan over medium-low heat and toss in the cumin seeds. Fry the seeds until they turn golden brown and release their aroma. Pour into the soup and immediately cover to allow the seasonings to steep into the hot dal for 1 to 2 minutes.

6. Garnish with olive oil, minced herbs, and pepper. Serve hot with the lime slices.

NOTES

- To make the soup in a pressure cooker, reduce the water to 3 cups; bring the soup up to pressure after adding all the ingredients in Step 2 and cook for 8 minutes.

- To make the soup in a slow cooker, put all the ingredients except the garnishes in a slow cooker and cook on high for about 3 hours.

VARIATIONS

- You can try this recipe with red lentils or whole mung beans (soak them for at least 8 hours).

- An equal amount of red lentils and yellow split mung dal is my favorite variation.

- Add 1 cup diced vegetables in Step 3 after the water comes to a boil.

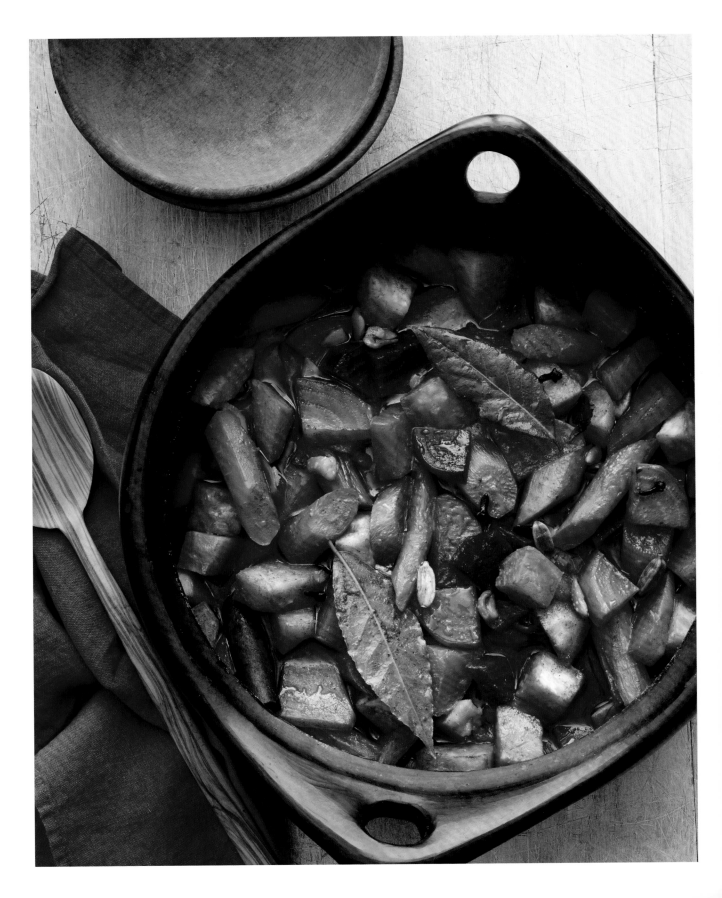

BRAISED ROOT VEGETABLES

PREP: 10 MINUTES (WITH ALREADY MADE WINTER VEGETABLE STOCK) ▪
COOK: ABOUT 60 MINUTES

serves 4 `GF` `DF`

Cooks in eighteenth-century France invented the braising method of cooking by putting coals under and atop the pot. Today we can achieve the same effect with an oven. What better way to "ground" yourself than to eat more root vegetables, which carry strong earthy energy! I find a moist, tender braise very balancing for when I feel Airy, especially on a cold day. Even though this dish takes at least an hour to cook, it is very low maintenance—it doesn't even require stirring while it's in the oven—so you can do something else in the meantime. Feel free to experiment with different combinations of root vegetables.

Experience the comfort of Braised Root Vegetables in the company of Einkorn Barley Biscuits (page 159) or Spiced Amaranth (page 149) and Cilantro Chutney (page 191).

1 tablespoon ghee or olive oil

4 cardamom pods

6 whole cloves

1-inch cinnamon stick

1 teaspoon ground coriander or Grounding Masala (page 222)

⅛ teaspoon asafoetida (optional)

⅓ cup cashews (whole or pieces) or blanched almonds (optional)

1 teaspoon salt

2 medium carrots, peeled and cut into 2-inch pieces (an oblique or diagonal cut looks beautiful in this dish)

1 small rutabaga, peeled, quartered, and cut into 1½-inch pieces (about 1 cup)

1 small red or golden beet, peeled, quartered, and sliced (about ½ cup)

½ cup daikon radish, cut into ½-inch-thick rounds

2 or 3 taro roots, peeled and cut into 2-inch cubes (about 1 cup)

½ cup peeled and cubed (1½-inch cubes) celery root

1 cup Winter Vegetable Stock (page 161), plus more if needed

2 bay leaves

3 sprigs fresh parsley or dill

GARNISH

2 tablespoons fresh herbs such as cilantro leaves or chopped dill or parsley

FOR FIERY DIGESTION: Use blanched almonds (not cashews); substitute 1 small zucchini or fennel for the beet and turnip.

FOR EARTHY DIGESTION: Replace the beets and carrots with a combination of either cauliflower or broccoli florets and chopped green cabbage or halved Brussels sprouts. Add 1 or 2 green seeded and minced Thai chiles with the spices in Step 2.

1. Preheat the oven to 350°F.

2. Heat the ghee in a Dutch oven, clay pot (stovetop and ovenproof), or ovenproof sauté pan over medium-low heat. Add the cardamom, cloves, and cinnamon and toast for 10 seconds, then add the coriander, asafoetida, and cashews and cook for 2 to 3 minutes, until the cashews brown slightly. Add the salt, carrots, rutabaga, beet, daikon, taro roots, and celery root, increase the heat to medium-high, and stir-fry for 3 to 4 minutes to slightly brown the vegetables. Pour in

vegetable stock to cover the vegetables by half and bring to a full boil. Top the vegetables with the bay leaves and parsley and turn off the heat.

3. Cover the pan with a tight-fitting lid and transfer to the oven. Braise the vegetables for 40 to 60 minutes, until they are very tender. Remove and discard the cinnamon stick, cardamom pods, bay leaves, and parley sprigs.

4. Garnish with the fresh herbs and serve hot.

NOTES

- To braise in a slow cooker, cook on low for 6 to 8 hours or overnight.

- To braise on the stovetop, in Step 2, continue to simmer the vegetables on the lowest heat without opening the lid for 30 minutes. Although faster, this method does not produce the same flavor and heartiness as braising the vegetables in the oven.

The Healing Benefits of Taro Root

Taro (*Colocasia esculenta*) is a root vegetable that resembles a hairy potato. It is used in many cuisines throughout the world, and it even grows as a decorative plant in the city gardens of New York. You can use taro as a potato substitute for almost any recipe. Taro surpasses potato in taste, nutrition, and medicinal benefits, and it is highly valued in Ayurveda as a prebiotic food (meaning it nourishes the friendly bacteria in the gut). With its slippery nature, taro serves as the "packaging and shipping" of toxins—it binds them in the colon and drives them out of the body, making it an important ingredient in detox Ayurvedic protocols. Taro is also very effective in soothing irritated stomach and gut. Other names for taro are albi, dasheen, eddo, and arbi.

SPINACH AND TARO SOUP

PREP: 5 MINUTES ▪ **COOK:** 20 MINUTES   serves 3 to 4 GF DF

This simple and calming soup supports recovery and builds strength. Eating it feels like giving yourself a "food hug."

Taro root is available in Indian and Asian grocery stores. It is best to use only the young taros (not bigger than a fist). Always peel and cook the taro; if eaten raw, taro can cause intense irritation.

2 or 3 taro roots, peeled and diced (1½ cups)

2 teaspoons ghee or olive oil

½ teaspoon salt

¼ teaspoon ground turmeric

5 ounces baby spinach or 1 pound bunched spinach, washed, stems removed, and chopped

2 teaspoons coriander seeds

½ teaspoon cumin seeds

⅛ teaspoon black peppercorns

GARNISHES

1 teaspoon olive oil

2 teaspoons fresh lime juice, or to taste

FOR FIERY DIGESTION: Omit the black pepper.

FOR EARTHY DIGESTION: Add 2 teaspoons grated fresh ginger or ½ teaspoon powdered ginger and omit the ghee or oil in Step 1.

1. In a 2-quart saucepan, bring 3 cups water to a boil over high heat. Add the taro root, ghee, salt, and turmeric. Reduce the heat to medium-low, cover, and simmer for 7 to 10 minutes, until the taro root is cooked through.

2. Add the spinach, stir, and cook covered for another 2 to 3 minutes, until the leaves wilt but remain vibrant green.

3. Turn off the heat. Uncover and let the soup cool down for a few minutes. Blend to a chunky or smooth consistency.

4. In a small skillet, dry-toast the coriander seeds, cumin seeds, and black peppercorns over low heat until they release their aroma and turn a shade darker. Grind to a fine powder in a spice grinder. Add spices to the soup (re-heat if necessary) and garnish with the olive oil and lime juice. Serve hot.

MIXED VEGETABLE CURRY IN CASHEW SAUCE

SOAK: OVERNIGHT ▪ **PREP:** 10 MINUTES ▪ **COOK:** 20 TO 25 MINUTES

serves 4 `GF` `DF`

"Is curry powder dried and ground curry leaves?" students often ask me in class. The answer is "No!" Curry powder is a spice blend for cooking curries. Curry leaves come from the curry tree and can be purchased in Indian or Asian grocery stores. The leaves will keep for up to two weeks if you store them refrigerated in an airtight container. Dried curry leaves are significantly less fragrant, so if that's all you have, double their quantity in a recipe.

In my early days of cooking, I used to finish curried vegetables with sour cream sauces, but then I realized how taxing this combination was for digestion. Soaked cashews creamed with a little water makes a lighter, dairy-free substitute for sour cream. The butter-soft cooked taro root also adds creaminess to the curry texture. This colorful Indian-style recipe is very adaptable. You can vary the combination of vegetables according to taste and availability—try summer squash, asparagus, Brussels sprouts, peas, sweet potatoes, broccoli, or whatever vegetables you have left in the fridge before your next shopping trip. Alternatively, you can roast some of the vegetables and add them when the rest of the vegetables are almost cooked. This curry goes well with Basmati Rice and Red Quinoa (page 101) or Cooling Basmati Rice (page 102) and Raisin-Cranberry Sauce (page 189) or Cilantro Chutney (page 191).

¼ cup cashews, soaked overnight, drained, and rinsed

2 tablespoons ghee or coconut oil

1 teaspoon ground turmeric

½ teaspoon cumin seeds

8 curry leaves

2 teaspoons minced fresh ginger

1 small green Thai chile, seeded and minced

1 teaspoon ground coriander

½ teaspoon dried thyme or rosemary (crushed)

⅛ teaspoon asafoetida (optional)

1½ teaspoons salt

3 medium taro roots, peeled and cut into ½-inch cubes

1 cup cubed (½-inch cubes) carrots

1 cup chopped (2-inch pieces) green beans

1 cup cauliflower florets (1-inch florets)

2 packed cups chopped spinach

GARNISH

2 tablespoons chopped fresh cilantro or parsley

FOR FIERY DIGESTION: Skip Step 1 and substitute coconut milk (page 217) for the cashew milk. Replace the ginger, chile, and asafoetida with ½ teaspoon Cooling Pungent Masala (page 222) in Step 2.

FOR EARTHY DIGESTION: Increase the ginger to 1 tablespoon and add one more green chile in Step 2.

1. Rinse the soaked cashews and blend them with 1½ cups water to a smooth cashew milk.

2. Heat the ghee in a 2-quart sauté pan over medium-low heat. Add the turmeric and toast for 15 seconds, then add the cumin seeds and continue to toast for a few more seconds, until the seeds darken a shade and release their aroma. Add the curry leaves, ginger,

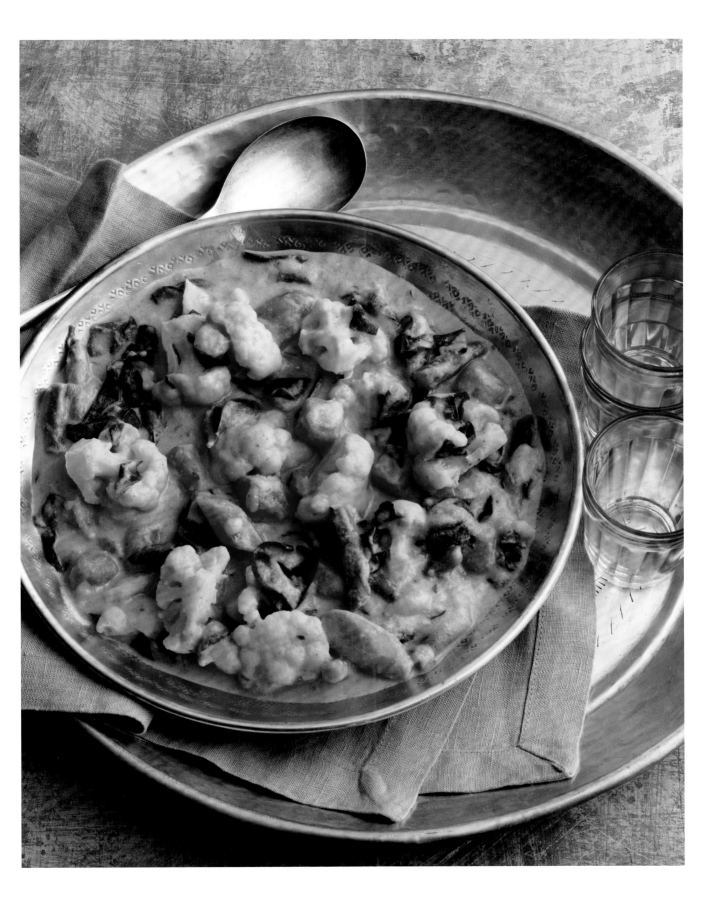

and chile and toast for a few more seconds, then add the coriander, thyme, asafoetida, if using, and salt. Immediately add the cashew milk and bring to a boil. Add the taro roots, cover, reduce the heat to medium-low, and simmer for 10 minutes. Add the carrots, green beans, and cauliflower, mix well, and continue to cook, covered, stirring occasionally, until the vegetables are tender, about 20 minutes. If the curry begins to dry and stick to the bottom of the pan, add ¼ cup more water. Add the spinach and cook for 5 more minutes. Add a little water if you like your curry more liquid.

3. Fold in the chopped fresh herbs and serve hot.

VARIATION

- Substitute ½ cup coconut milk (page 217) for the cashew milk.

The Healing Benefits of Curry Leaves

Leaves from the tropical curry tree (*Murraya koenigii* or *Bergera koenigii*) are also called sweet neem leaves in India. Their unique bittersweet aroma attracts cooks across the globe, but it is the numerous healing benefits that elevate curry leaves to an herbal tonic for daily cooking. I've been home-raising a small curry tree in our apartment in New York City for several years now. It not only supplies me with leaves for cooking, but it also beautifies the room and purifies the air. Here are a few of the important medicinal properties of curry leaves:

- Support liver detoxification

- Purify the blood

- Reduce bad cholesterol

- Are anti-diabetic

- Fight microorganisms in the gut

- Enhance digestion and absorption

- Nourish the hair

- Alleviate burns and bruises when used as a poultice

- Help with morning sickness

KALE AND ROASTED SWEET POTATOES

PREP: 5 TO 10 MINUTES ▪ **COOK:** ABOUT 30 MINUTES   serves 4 `GF` `DF`

I love the green-orange autumn colors, texture contrasts, grounding flavors, and simple preparation of this dish. In it, I balance the bitter, cooling, and light qualities of kale with warming spices and the density and heaviness of roasted sweet potato so that you can enjoy this nutrient-rich leafy green even on a cold, windy day.

1 medium sweet potato, peeled and cubed (1½-inch cubes; about 2 cups)

2 tablespoons melted ghee, sesame oil, or olive oil

2 teaspoons thinly julienned fresh ginger

⅛ teaspoon asafoetida (optional)

1 teaspoon Digestive Masala (page 223) or Grounding Masala (page 222)

¼ teaspoon freshly ground black pepper

¼ teaspoon salt

1 bunch kale (1½ pounds), stemmed and torn into 2-inch pieces (5 packed cups/about ½ pound)

GARNISHES

2 teaspoons olive oil

Sprinkle of fresh lime juice

FOR FIERY DIGESTION: Omit the ginger, asafoetida, and black pepper; substitute Superspice Masala (page 219) or Cooling Masala (page 222) for the Digestive Masala.

FOR EARTHY DIGESTION: Substitute Energizing Masala (page 221) for the Digestive Masala; reduce the sweet potato to 1 cup and increase the chopped kale to 6 to 7 cups.

1. Preheat the oven to 400°F.

2. Place the sweet potatoes in a small baking dish, drizzle with 1 tablespoon melted ghee, and mix to coat it in the ghee. Bake until the cubes are soft with a slightly golden crust, about 25 minutes.

3. Heat a large skillet over medium-low heat and add the remaining 1 tablespoon ghee. Add the ginger and toast for about 15 seconds, until the ginger strips brown slightly, then add the asafoetida, if using, masala, the black pepper, salt, and kale. Use salad tongs to mix well, then cover and cook for 2 to 3 minutes, until the kale wilts. Stir again—if the kale is too dry and begins to stick to the pot, add a tablespoon of water. The kale is done when it is soft and succulent yet vibrant green. Garnish the kale with olive oil and lime juice.

4. Serve the roasted sweet potatoes hot on a bed of sautéed kale.

VARIATION

▪ Replace the kale with other greens, such as collards, spinach, beet greens, or chard. Replace the sweet potatoes with beets, celery root, carrots, or turnips.

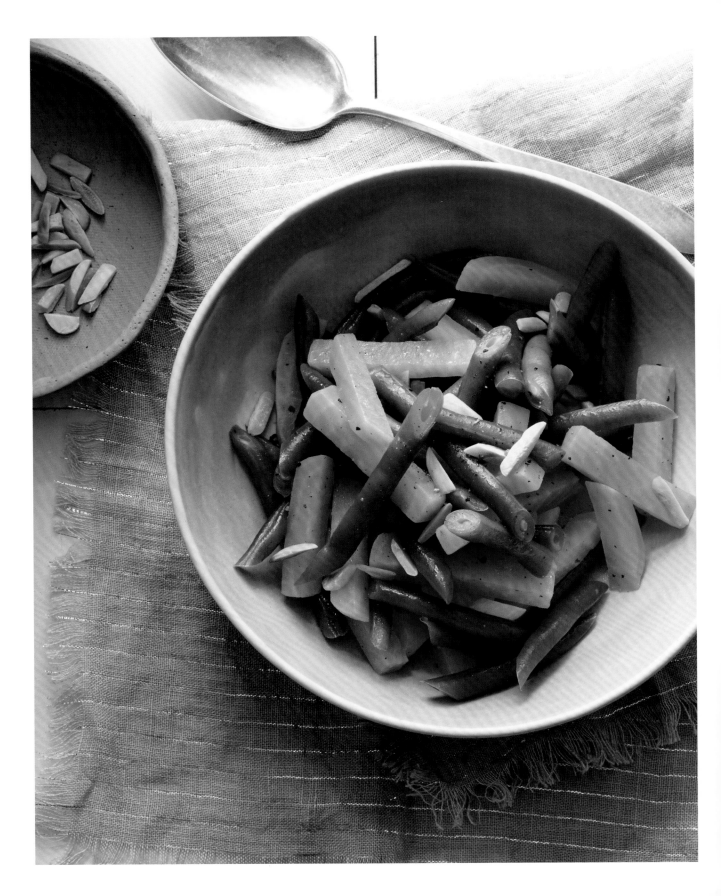

GOLDEN BEET AND GREEN BEAN SALAD

PREP: 10 MINUTES ■ **COOK:** 15 MINUTES   serves 4 `GF` `DF`

Raw salads really go against the law of balance when you want to warm up or when you're experiencing Airy digestion. Raw foods, being cold and rough by nature, need strong digestive fire to "cook" in the stomach. If balance is your aim, go for cooked salads in fall and winter. Blanching is a great cooking technique if you really want a crisp salad in the winter but you prefer to avoid raw foods.

1 teaspoon salt

2 or 3 medium golden beets, cut into ¼-inch-wide and 2-inch-long pieces (2 cups)

2 cups green beans or French beans, end trimmed and cut into 2-inch pieces

1 tablespoon olive oil

Small pinch of asafoetida

¼ teaspoon freshly ground black pepper

1 tablespoon fresh lime juice

2 teaspoons ginger juice (see Note)

GARNISHES

¼ cup toasted slivered almonds or pecan halves (optional)

2 tablespoons sliced (cut into thin ribbons) opal or regular basil leaves

FOR FIERY DIGESTION: Omit the asafoetida. Reduce or omit the black pepper.

FOR EARTHY DIGESTION: Add more black pepper to taste. Substitute peeled and sliced sunchokes for the beets if you like.

1. Prepare a bowl for refreshing the blanched vegetables by filling it up halfway with cold water and adding a handful of ice.

2. To blanch the vegetables, fill a 3- to 4-quart saucepan halfway with water, cover, and bring to a full boil over high heat; add ½ teaspoon of the salt. Add the beets and cook for 5 minutes, or until they are tender. Use a slotted spoon to transfer the beets from the boiling water to the bowl of iced water and refresh the vegetables in it for 10 seconds, then transfer to a mesh strainer. Repeat with the green beans (make sure the water is rapidly boiling again before adding them). Drain the vegetables well, then transfer them to a serving dish. You can reserve the hot blanching water for cooking a soup, stock, or curry if you like.

3. In a small pan or a metal measuring cup, slightly heat the olive oil over low heat, then add the asafoetida and pepper and toast for 5 seconds.

4. In a small bowl, whisk together the infused olive oil, the lime juice, ginger juice, and remaining ½ teaspoon salt. Pour the dressing over the vegetables and gently toss.

5. Serve at room temperature garnished with the toasted nuts and basil.

NOTE

■ To make ginger juice, grate a 1½-inch piece of ginger and squeeze to release its juice with your hand.

APPLE MUFFINS

PREP: 10 TO 15 MINUTES ▪ **BAKE:** 15 TO 20 MINUTES   makes 9 muffins GF DF

"Heaven shaped in the form of a muffin." These were the words of my friend and bestselling author Donna LeBlanc when she first made and tasted these in one of my cooking classes. Grounding yet light and moist, Apple Muffins satisfy everyone's craving for something sweet. They go well with a hot beverage.

½ cup Ayurvedic buttermilk (page 213)
   or water

⅔ cup Sucanat or raw cane sugar

¼ cup melted ghee or coconut oil

1 tablespoon fresh lime juice

2 cups whole einkorn flour (206 grams)

1½ teaspoons Sweet Masala (page 220)
   or 1 teaspoon ground cinnamon
   plus ½ teaspoon ground cardamom

1¼ teaspoons baking powder

½ teaspoon baking soda

¼ teaspoon salt

1 large apple, peeled and grated (1½ cups)

¼ cup chopped walnuts or pecans (optional)

FOR FIERY DIGESTION: Enjoy the muffins as they are.

FOR EARTHY DIGESTION: Use 1 cup (120 grams) barley flour plus ⅔ cup (69 grams) einkorn flour and omit the nuts.

1. Place an oven rack in the center of the oven and preheat the oven to 400°F. Line a muffin pan with unbleached paper cups.

2. In a small saucepan, slightly warm the buttermilk over low heat (it should not be hot).

Turn off the heat and whisk in the Sucanat, ghee, and lime juice.

3. In a medium bowl, mix the flour, masala, baking powder, baking soda, and salt.

4. Fold the liquid ingredients into the dry ingredients, stirring a few times with a light touch, just enough to create a soft batter. (Overmixing develops the gluten and makes the muffins stiff.)

5. Fold in the apples and walnuts.

6. Spoon the batter into the muffin cups three-quarters of the way up. Bake for 15 to 20 minutes, until golden brown.

7. Let the muffins cool in the pan for 5 minutes, then transfer to a cooling rack. Serve warm or at room temperature.

NOTE

▪ **Gluten-free option:** Substitute 1⅔ cups (228 grams) sorghum flour, ⅓ cup (40 grams) amaranth flour, and 2 tablespoons arrowroot powder for the einkorn flour; add ¼ cup water in Step 2. Use paper cups for baking, as gluten-free muffins are more crumbly.

CARROT-WALNUT CAKE

PREP: 10 MINUTES ▪ **BAKE:** ABOUT 30 MINUTES   serves 8 DF

No dairy and no eggs, but rich in flavor, soft in texture, and most delectable: this cake in a nut-shell. The coconut sugar contributes to rich brown color, darker than the usual carrot cake.

For complete enjoyment, serve Carrot-Walnut Cake with Almond Milk Chai (page 181), Ginger Mint Limeade (page 89), or Rose Tea (page 133).

1¾ cups (185 grams) whole einkorn or
   1½ cup (165 grams) sifted spelt flour

¼ cup arrowroot powder

2 tablespoons ground cinnamon

½ teaspoon ground nutmeg

1 teaspoon baking powder

¼ teaspoon baking soda

¼ teaspoon salt

1 cup grated carrots

½ cup chopped walnuts or pecans

¼ cup maple syrup

¼ cup coconut sugar

½ cup raw applesauce (see Note)

2 tablespoons fresh orange juice or lime juice

1 teaspoon vanilla extract

½ cup raisins

½ cup melted coconut oil

DECORATION

8 toasted walnut halves

Thinly grated orange zest (optional)

FOR FIERY DIGESTION: Enjoy as is.

FOR EARTHY DIGESTION: Add 1 tablespoon ginger juice (grate a 2-inch piece of ginger and squeeze out the juice with your hand) to the wet ingredients in Step 3.

1. Preheat the oven to 350°F. Grease a 9-inch cake pan or 7 x 12 x ¾-inch jellyroll pan and dust with flour.

2. In a large bowl, whisk together the flour, arrowroot, cinnamon, nutmeg, baking powder, baking soda, and salt. Fold in the carrots and walnuts.

3. In a separate bowl, whisk together the maple syrup, coconut sugar, applesauce, orange juice, vanilla, raisins, and coconut oil.

4. Fold the wet ingredients into the dry ingredients; stir only as much as needed to combine all the ingredients (overmixing will make your cake stiff).

5. Pour the batter into the prepared pan and bake for 30 minutes, or until a toothpick or skewer inserted in the middle of the cake comes out clean.

6. Let the cake cool in the pan before cutting. Decorate each piece with toasted walnut halves or orange zest.

NOTE

▪ To make raw applesauce, peel and chop an apple and puree it in a small food processor or blender until smooth.

DATE AND NUT TEA BISCUITS

PREP: 5 MINUTES ▪ **BAKE:** 15 MINUTES   makes about 15 tea biscuits `GF` `DF`

I really wanted to include a cookie recipe in this book. Not that we need cookies to stay healthy, but sometimes, especially around holidays, we deserve a little extra pleasure. My philosophy is, if I'm going to eat cookies, they'd better be as healthy as possible. Note that these buttery, crumbly tea biscuits do not expand during baking.

1 cup (109 grams) einkorn or ¾ cup (81 grams) spelt flour

⅔ cup ground hazelnuts, almonds, or finely shredded coconut

1 teaspoon Sweet Masala (page 220)

½ teaspoon baking powder

Small pinch of salt

⅓ cup ghee, coconut oil, or unsalted cultured butter (soft but not melted)

½ cup finely chopped dates, soaked in hot water for 5 minutes and drained

½ teaspoon vanilla extract

> **FOR FIERY DIGESTION:** Enjoy these as they are.
>
> **FOR EARTHY DIGESTION:** Take a little bite, but don't indulge—as addictive as these cookies are, they are too heavy and fattening for you.

1. In a medium bowl, whisk together the flour, nuts, masala, baking powder, and salt.

2. In a food processor, beat the ghee, dates, and vanilla to a paste.

3. Add the dry mixture to the date mixture in the food processor and pulse a few times, until the ingredients are well incorporated.

4. Preheat the oven to 350°F. Grease a baking sheet or line it with parchment paper.

5. Roll the dough into 1-inch balls, flatten them to about ⅓-inch thick, and place on the baking sheet about 1 inch apart. You may also roll out the dough with a rolling pin to about ⅓-inch thick and shape the cookies with a cookie cutter.

6. Bake for 13 to 15 minutes, until the tea biscuits develop a thin crust. When you take the cookies out of the oven, they will still be soft, but don't worry—they will harden as they cool.

7. Transfer the tea biscuits to a wire rack and let them cool before serving.

NOTES

- Before placing the cookies in the oven, you may decorate them with some chopped or sliced nuts.

- Gluten-free option: Substitute ½ cup teff flour (60 grams) and ½ cup arrowroot powder (64 grams) for the einkorn flour; add ¼ cup almond milk (page 216) in Step 2. Bake at 375°F for 18 minutes.

CLOCKWISE FROM TOP LEFT: Almond Milk Chai, Carrot-Walnut Cake, Date and Nut Tea Biscuits

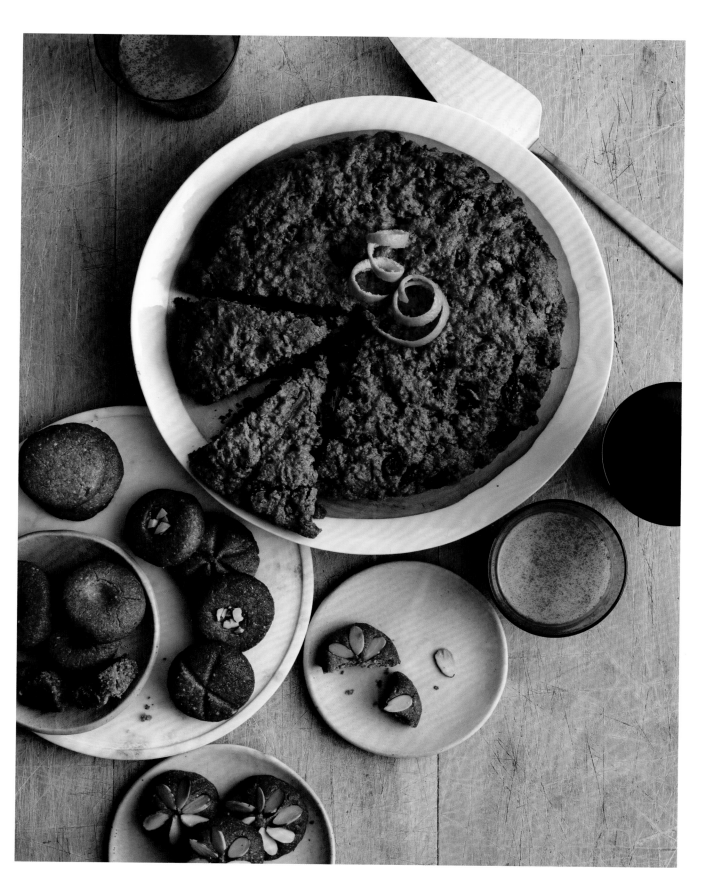

GROUNDING DIGESTIVE TEA

PREP: 10 MINUTES

serves 2

I've seen many different variations of this famous recipe for Ayurvedic digestive tea made with fennel, cumin, and coriander, but I wanted to share my favorite one. It offers great comfort to the stomach and eliminates gas, burping, and bloating.

I included this recipe in the Airy chapter, but Digestive Tea is good to drink every day, whether you're feeling Airy, Fiery, or Earthy. Sipping a cup (no more) of this tea will moisten drier foods and enhance digestion, especially at lunchtime. You could also drink it an hour after a meal. One of the worst eating habits is drinking a glass of cold water or ice-cold beverage at the end of your meal. What happens when you pour water on fire? You guessed it: your digestive fire will diminish.

2 cups boiling hot water

½ teaspoon fennel seeds

½ teaspoon coriander seeds

½ teaspoon cumin seeds

In a small saucepan or teapot, pour the hot water over the seeds, cover, and steep for 10 minutes. Strain, let the tea cool a little, and sip slowly.

ALMOND MILK CHAI

COOK: 30 MINUTES

serves 2 to 3 GF DF

When I lived in India, I learned that chai is one of those "as many cooks, as many recipes" dishes. The variations are countless. I can still hear the train vendors' loud and yowling cries of *"Chaaaiiii,"* but I could never produce the same exact incantation.

    Chai means "tea" in Hindi. This recipe is my caffeine-free version of a traditional SV Ayurvedic masala chai that helps us digest carbohydrates and transform sugar into energy. It is especially good to drink when you want to counteract the effects of eating sweets. The almond milk is essential for balancing the pungent spices.

10 black peppercorns

5 cardamom pods, crushed

5 whole cloves

1 tablespoon grated fresh ginger

1½ cinnamon sticks

1 star anise (optional)

2 tablespoons raw sugar or sweetener of
    your choice, or to taste (optional)

1 cup almond milk (page 216)

FOR FIERY DIGESTION: Omit the black pepper. Reduce the ginger to 1 teaspoon; add 1 teaspoon coriander seeds and 5 fresh mint leaves in Step 1.

FOR EARTHY DIGESTION: Increase the ginger to 1½ teaspoons; add 1 teaspoon dried gymnema leaf (see Notes) and steep it for 5 minutes after turning off the heat and before straining in Step 1. Cool the tea down a little and sweeten with 1 teaspoon honey.

1. Bring 4 cups water to a full boil, then add the peppercorns, cardamom, cloves, ginger, cinnamon, and star anise. Reduce the heat to medium-low, cover, and brew for 30 minutes. Strain the chai, add the sugar, and stir well to dissolve it.

2. Let the chai sit uncovered for 5 minutes to cool it down a bit, then stir in the almond milk. Serve hot.

NOTES

- You can substitute whole milk for the almond milk; add it to the pot 20 minutes into cooking.

- If scaling up the recipe by more than triple, reduce the spices by one third.

- Gymnema leaf is a bitter herb known for its ability to improve sugar metabolism.

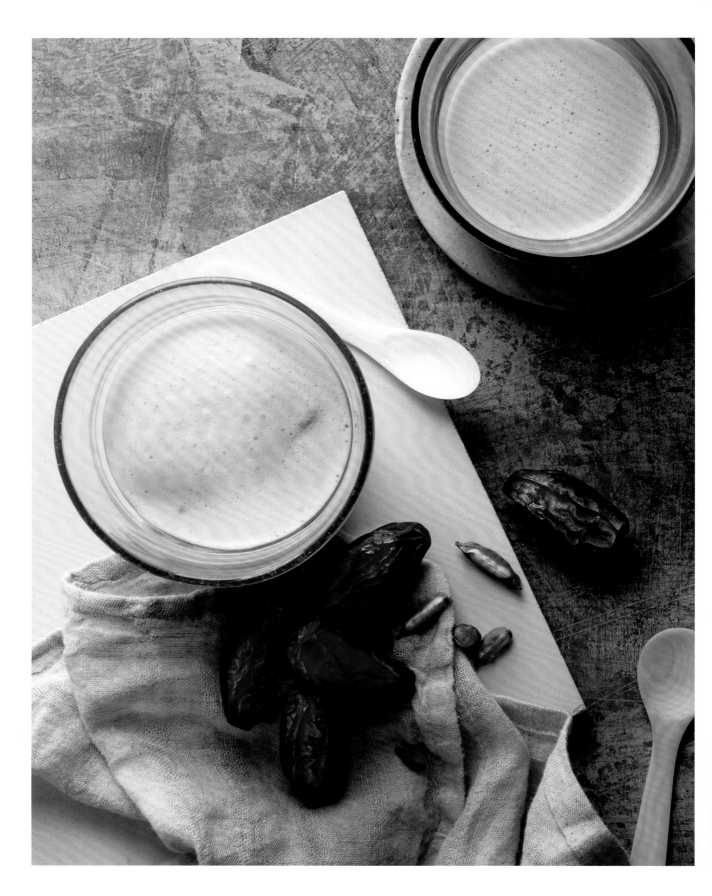

CALMING DATE MILKSHAKE

COOK: 10 MINUTES

serves 1 GF DF

As the day wanes, the moon rises and rules the night with its cooling and calming energy. This is the ideal time for us to shift gears from dynamism to restful sleep—the perfect balance between action and inaction. Unfortunately, we may often find ourselves stretching work or socializing past 9 p.m., thus straining our nervous system and disrupting the built-in rhythms of the body and mind designed to detoxify and recharge.

If you feel high-strung and tired but unable to fall asleep or stay asleep at night, try this milkshake (drink it on its own). It is a classic SV Ayurvedic recipe to help us pacify the nervous system before bedtime, sleep through the night, and wake up energized. I also like to sip on Calming Date Milkshake when I feel a little hungry before going to bed but when it's too late to eat and digest a full meal. Enjoyed regularly, this milkshake will nourish and support your physiology in many ways: to reduce airiness, overcome fatigue, and gain weight (if you need it).

1 cup whole milk or almond milk (page 216)

3 cardamom pods, slightly crushed open on one end

1-inch cinnamon stick

1 or 2 Medjool dates, pitted and chopped

¼ teaspoon vanilla extract (optional)

FOR FIERY DIGESTION: Substitute ½ teaspoon Sweet Masala (page 220) for the cardamom and cinnamon. If you are very hungry, add 10 soaked and peeled almonds in Step 2.

FOR EARTHY DIGESTION: Substitute almond milk for the whole milk or dilute the whole milk with water by half.

1. In a small saucepan, combine the milk, cardamom, and cinnamon. Bring to a boil over medium-high heat, then reduce the heat and simmer uncovered for 10 minutes. Take it off the heat, remove the cardamom and cinnamon, and let the milk cool down a little.

2. Transfer to a blender, add the date and vanilla, and blend until smooth. Drink the milkshake warm or heat it up again and sip it hot.

SUGGESTED GROUNDING MENUS

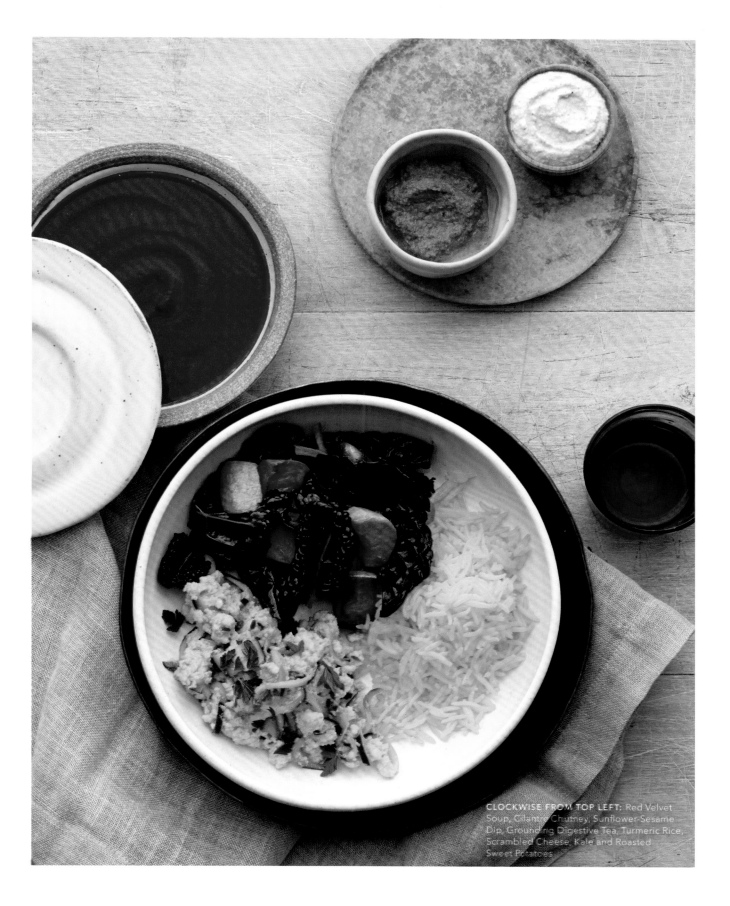

CLOCKWISE FROM TOP LEFT: Red Velvet Soup, Cilantro Chutney, Sunflower-Sesame Dip, Grounding Digestive Tea, Turmeric Rice, Scrambled Cheese, Kale and Roasted Sweet Potatoes

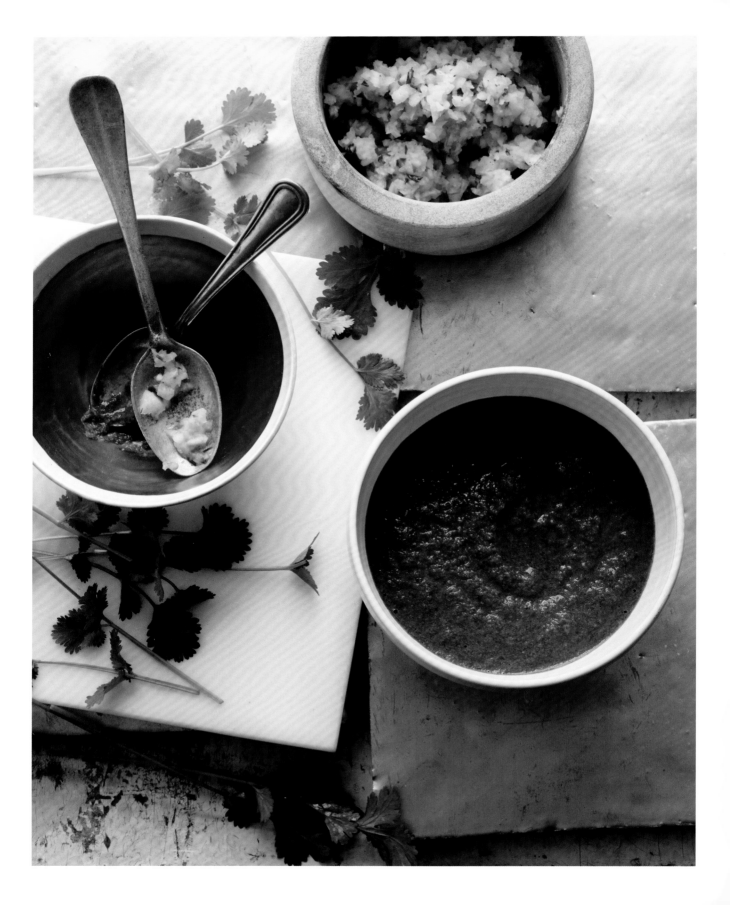

ACCOMPANIMENTS
&
SALAD
DRESSINGS

Dips, dressings, sauces, and toppings make plain vegetables or grains exciting and add a nuance of flavor and color to an elaborate meal. They also moisturize drier foods.

The recipes in this chapter are generally balancing for everyone unless I indicate otherwise in the headnote or specify variations for different types of digestion.

ALMOND MILK BÉCHAMEL SAUCE

COOK: 5 TO 10 MINUTES (WITH ALREADY MADE ALMOND MILK)   makes about 2 cups

I created this recipe years ago when I wanted to make lasagna with white sauce but I realized that milk and salt were incompatible for digestion according to Ayurveda. To create a lighter, more digestible version of the classic French sauce, I chose ghee or olive oil over butter, replaced the milk with almond milk, and used whole-grain flour. The result is marvelous.

I use Almond Milk Béchamel in Lasagna with Broccolini, Carrots, and Spinach (page 112), but you can serve it with steamed vegetables and even as a sauce for homemade pizza.

¼ cup ghee or olive oil

3½ tablespoons whole einkorn flour or spelt flour

2 cups almond milk (page 216)

¾ teaspoon salt

⅛ teaspoon asafoetida

¼ teaspoon ground nutmeg

¼ teaspoon ground white pepper

1 teaspoon Italian seasoning blend or ½ teaspoon dried basil plus ½ teaspoon dried oregano

1. Melt the ghee in a 2-quart sauté pan or saucier. Add the flour and toast for 1 minute, stirring constantly with a whisk to eliminate all lumps.

2. While stirring constantly, gradually add the almond milk and all of the seasonings. Bring to a simmer and continue to whisk constantly until the sauce begins to bubble; cook for about 2 minutes, until the sauce stops thickening. Keep in mind that the sauce will thicken more as it cools down.

NOTES

■ **Gluten-free option:** Substitute 4 tablespoons amaranth flour for the einkorn or spelt flour.

RAISIN-CRANBERRY SAUCE

COOK: 20 TO 25 MINUTES   serves 6 to 8 (makes 1½ cups) `GF` `DF`

This sauce looks like and tastes like barbecue sauce (or even better) without any tomato in it. When blended together, the underlying smoky flavor of black cardamom and the supporting flavors of the rest of the spices round up the tart and astringent cranberries and sweet raisins perfectly. You can enjoy a color, consistency, and taste similar to that of tomato ketchup, making this sauce a nice substitute for those of us who prefer to avoid tomatoes in their diet.

As piquant as this sauce is, I do not advise eating it every day because of the heavy acid content of the cranberries. With its deep red color and a medley of all six tastes, Raisin-Cranberry Sauce goes well with the Skillet Vegetable Pie (page 81), Scrambled Cheese (page 151), Quinoa Flakes and Vegetable Upma (page 99), and many other dishes.

½ teaspoon cumin seeds

⅛ teaspoon black peppercorns

¾ cup dried cranberries

1 tablespoon olive oil

4 black cardamom pods, slightly crushed on one end but not fully opened

2 green Thai chiles, seeded (no need to chop)

1 bay leaf or 4 curry leaves

¾ to 1 teaspoon salt

½ teaspoon Digestive Masala (page 223)

½ cup golden raisins

¼ cup Thompson raisins or 5 dried pitted prunes

1 teaspoon fresh lime juice

FOR AIRY DIGESTION: Enjoy as is.

FOR FIERY DIGESTION: Avoid this sauce, especially if you have acidic digestion—the cranberries will be too sour for you. If you don't have hyperacidity, then enjoy a tablespoon of this sauce without the chiles.

FOR EARTHY DIGESTION: Enjoy as is or add one more chile for extra pungency.

1. Grind the cumin seeds and peppercorns to a powder—a mortar and pestle will work well here, or use a spice grinder.

2. In a small saucepan, combine 1½ cups water, the ground cumin and pepper, the cranberries, olive oil, black cardamom, chiles, bay leaf, salt, and masala. Place over medium-high heat, bring to a gentle boil, then reduce the heat and cook uncovered for 10 minutes. Add both types of raisins and continue to simmer for another 10 to 15 minutes, until the cranberries become mushy and the raisins are soft and plump. Set aside uncovered to cool down a bit.

3. Remove the black cardamom pods and bay leaf. Transfer to a blender and blend until smooth.

4. Transfer to a serving dish and stir in the lime juice. Serve warm or at room temperature.

5. The sauce will keep in an airtight container in the refrigerator for up to 3 days.

KALE AND ARUGULA PESTO

PREP: 10 TO 15 MINUTES   makes about 1 cup **GF** **DF**

I think basil is one of the herbs that keeps Italian food lovers healthy despite that cuisine's heavy pastas and cheeses. Adding basil does more than create an appetizing taste and aroma; the herb is a powerful digestive aid that keeps your circulatory channels open. This pesto is very nutritious, and sautéing the kale and arugula makes them friendlier to the stomach.

This emerald-green sauce goes well with Lasagna with Broccolini, Carrots, and Spinach (page 112), Spinach Risotto (page 111), and Steamed Artichokes with Olive Tapenade (page 125), but you don't have to limit its pleasures to Italian-themed menus. Why not top steamed vegetables or fold fresh cheese cubes into it?

4 ounces kale leaves, washed, stemmed, and coarsely chopped

½ cup olive oil

¼ teaspoon asafoetida (optional)

2 packed cups baby arugula

1 cup toasted and coarsely chopped walnuts

¼ packed cup chopped fresh basil leaves

2 tablespoons water

1 tablespoon fresh lime juice

1 teaspoon salt, or to taste

½ teaspoon cracked black pepper

1. Pulse the kale leaves in a food processor until minced—they should now measure 2 cups.

2. In a large sauté pan, lightly heat the olive oil over medium-low heat. Add the asafoetida, if using, then the minced kale and baby arugula and stir for a minute or two for the greens to wilt and absorb the oil.

3. Return the greens to the food processor (no need to wash it in between steps), add the walnuts, basil, water, lime juice, salt, and pepper and pulse to a rough paste. (I prefer it more on the chunky than smooth side.)

4. To store, transfer to a closed container and refrigerate for up to a week.

CILANTRO CHUTNEY

PREP: 5 TO 10 MINUTES

makes ½ cup `GF` `DF`

This chutney and its variations are my favorites for improving any type of indigestion. Cilantro is a super food and a heavy metal detoxifier, but it's hard to get enough of it just as a garnish. Blending this potent herb into chutney is a delectable way to eat more.

You can serve this bright-green sauce as a digestive aid with every meal. It will freshen up and invigorate basically everything savory: lentil soups, grains, vegetables, breads, cutlets. If possible, make the chutney just before serving, as its flavors and healing properties fade with time, even if refrigerated. The recommended serving is 2 to 3 tablespoons per person.

2½ cups coarsely chopped packed cilantro with stems

2 tablespoons fresh lime juice

2 tablespoons water

1 tablespoon peeled and minced fresh ginger

1 green Thai chile, seeded

1 teaspoon honey, maple syrup, or a pitted chopped date

½ teaspoon salt

1 tablespoon olive oil

- ¼ cup soaked, blanched almonds or ¼ cup pulp from making almond milk

- ¼ cup shredded dried or fresh coconut

- ¼ cup soaked and drained cashews

- ¼ cup chopped avocado

- ½ teaspoon toasted Superspice Masala (page 219)

- Fully or partially chopped mint (hard stems removed) instead of the cilantro (for those who cannot tolerate the taste of cilantro)

FOR FIERY DIGESTION: Reduce the fresh ginger to 1 teaspoon or replace it with ½ teaspoon powdered sunthi ginger (see page 89); omit the green chile and sweetener.

In a blender, combine all the ingredients except the olive oil and blend to a creamy sauce. Add the olive oil and briefly pulse to mix it in. To store, refrigerate in a covered container for up to 24 hours.

VARIATIONS

- Try one of these add-ins (adjust salt to taste and water to a creamy sauce consistency):

- ¼ cup coconut milk (page 217)

The Healing Benefits of Cilantro

With its sweet, pungent, astringent taste and cooling effect, cilantro is always balancing no matter how you feel. It also:

- Strengthens digestion

- Calms hyperacidity in the stomach

- Relieves coughs and fever

- Acts as a powerful binder of environmental toxins, especially heavy metals

- Thins the blood

- Works as a mouth freshener

DAIKON RADISH CHUTNEY

My husband, Prentiss, loves this chutney. In his words, "The mustardy pungent taste grows on your palate after swallowing each bite." Fresh, crunchy, and with a gentle turmeric glow, this condiment will spice up any grain or vegetable. It is so good for your liver and kidneys that it is also suitable to include in cleansing protocols.

When discussing members of the radish family, Ayurveda recommends the rare icicle daikon or the more common long white radishes easily found in grocery stores. Make sure your radish is somewhat soft (the very hard ones are too mature) and is not thicker than 2 inches in diameter—thinner radishes are generally balancing for everyone, while the fat ones are aggravating for most people. If you only have red radishes on hand, you may substitute them for the daikon in this recipe.

2 teaspoons olive oil

½ teaspoon Digestive Masala (page 223)

1 cup peeled and diced daikon radish

1 tablespoon fresh lime juice

½ teaspoon salt

3 tablespoons coarsely chopped fresh cilantro or 2 tablespoons fresh mint leaves

1. In a metal measuring cup or a small pan, lightly heat the olive oil over low heat; add the masala and cook until it releases its aroma, 5 to 10 seconds.

2. Place the daikon, masala oil, and lime juice in a food processor and pulse a few times to achieve a flaky consistency. Scrape down the sides of the bowl, add the salt and cilantro, and pulse once or twice to incorporate them. Be careful: overblending will make your chutney too watery, with merged colors.

3. You may refrigerate this chutney in a closed container, but it is best to eat it immediately after making it because with time the daikon releases its sulfury aroma, which some people find repulsive.

The Healing Benefits of Daikon Radish

Thin daikon radish deserves the recognition it enjoyed from Ayurveda thousands of years ago. Although pungent and heating, because it pulls out hot toxins, daikon ultimately reduces acidity. It also:

- Calms the nervous system

- Supports digestion

- Reduces water retention

- Cleanses the kidneys, gallbladder, liver, blood, and eyes

- Relieves hemorrhoids

- Clears the vocal cords, making it great for singers and public speakers

- Eliminates catarrhal congestion in the body, especially in the sinuses

GOLDEN CHEESE CUBES

COOK: ABOUT 20 MINUTES (WITH ALREADY-PRESSED CHEESE)   makes 1 cup `GF`

Indian cuisine uses a lot of deep-fried cheese, but deep-frying makes food taxing for the liver, and restaurants often fry food in toxic hydrogenated, reused oil. You can give this cheese a beautiful golden crust by baking or pan-frying it. I like to brighten the cubes with a little turmeric; see photo on page 195–don't they look welcoming?

Golden Cheese Cubes add extra protein, color, texture, and grounding to any leafy greens and non-starchy vegetables or soups, so try them with Sautéed Leafy Greens (page 118), Broccoli Rabe and Cauliflower (page 70), or Green Cabbage and Kale (page 75). To add moisture, serve the cheese with Cilantro Chutney (page 191) or Raisin-Cranberry Sauce (page 189). You can also coat these golden cubes with Kale and Arugula Pesto (page 190) for an attractive appetizer.

5 ounces fresh pressed cheese (page 202)

1 teaspoon ghee

¼ teaspoon ground turmeric

¼ teaspoon salt

1. Preheat the oven to 350°F.

2. Cut the pressed cheese into 1½-inch cubes for a yield of 1 cup.

3. In a metal measuring cup or a small pan over low heat, melt the ghee with the turmeric and salt. Pour it over the cheese cubes and rub it in gently.

4. Spread the cheese cubes over a small baking pan such as an 8 x 8-inch Pyrex pan and bake until the cubes develop a slight golden crust, 20 to 25 minutes. Carefully toss the cubes with a spatula at least once while baking to prevent them from sticking to the pan.

5. Serve hot with vegetables or soup.

NOTES

- Instead of baking, you can pan-fry the cheese cubes in the ghee (add an extra tablespoon to prevent them from sticking to the pan). This method is best for when you're feeling Airy.

- If you're cubing the cheese in advance, keep the cheese cubes soaking in hot water until you're ready to make this recipe—the cheese will remain spongy and succulent.

TOASTED DULSE CHIPS

PREP: 5 MINUTES   makes 1 cup

These crunchy, glistening sea-vegetable chips promptly disappear from the dining table, no matter the quantity. Is it the salty taste, ocean flavor, or mineral-rich nutrition that tempts you to grab some more? People often ask me, "What is a good source of iodine and vitamin B12 for vegetarians?" Sea vegetables, folks! Please note that this dish may aggravate you if you're having Fiery digestion.

I like to serve these brown-maroon-colored chips with salads, grains, stir-fries, and stews. The chips lose their crunch once they touch moist food, so it's best to make them right before eating. Reduce or omit the salt in any dish they accompany.

1 cup whole-leaf dulse

1 teaspoon ghee or coconut oil

1. Tear the dulse leaves into bite-size pieces (try not to crumble them).

2. Melt the ghee in a small pan over medium heat. Add the dulse and, with the help of salad tongs, gently toss the leaves to coat them with ghee. Continue to toss until the dulse crisps into chips, 4 to 5 minutes, making sure the ghee doesn't start to smoke.

3. Transfer to a serving dish and serve promptly.

NOTE

■ Whole-leaf dulse is available in health food stores and Asian grocery stores. Eden and Emerald Cove are great brands.

FROM TOP: Golden Cheese Cubes, Toasted Dulse Chips

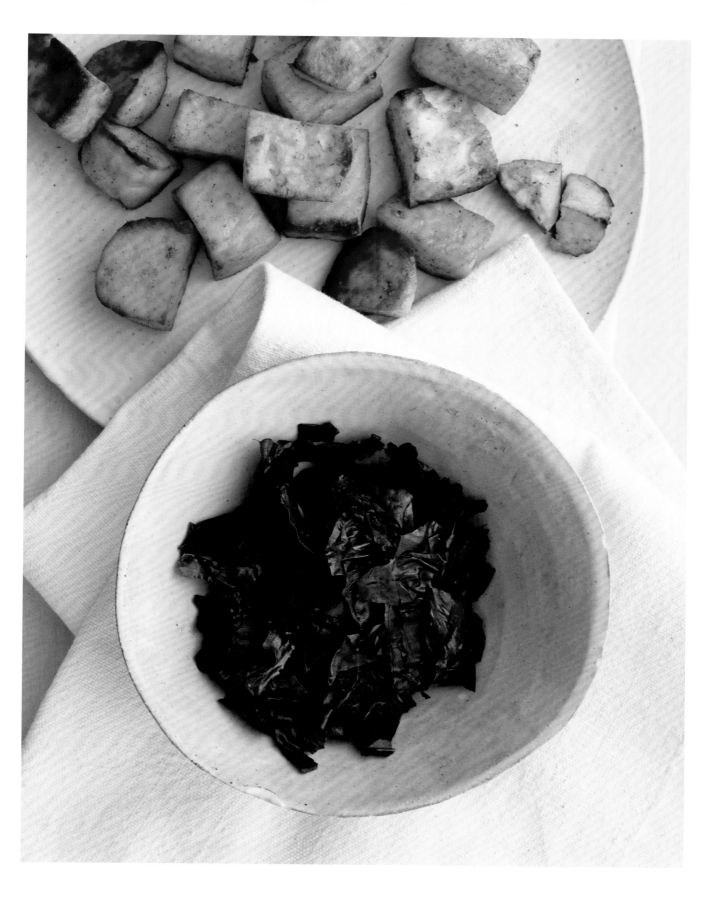

CREAMY CUCUMBER DRESSING

PREP: 5 TO 10 MINUTES

makes 1 cup

This dressing is so creamy that you'll never guess it is nut free and dairy free. The asafoetida and fresh herbs help make the sweet, heavy, and watery cucumber more digestible. Ayurveda lists cucumbers and lemons as incompatible when eaten together, so make sure to use limes here.

This cooling dressing is best with salads during the summer or as a sauce on top of steamed grains and vegetables.

¼ cup olive oil

⅛ teaspoon asafoetida (optional)

1 cup peeled and chopped cucumber (if the seeds are hard, scoop them out)

1½ tablespoons fresh lime juice

¾ teaspoon salt

1½ tablespoons minced fresh dill, basil, or parsley (or 1 teaspoon dried herb)

1. In a metal measuring cup or a small pan, heat the olive oil on the lowest heat, add the asafoetida, if using, and lightly toast until it releases its aroma, 5 to 10 seconds.

2. Pour the oil in to a blender, add the cucumber, lime juice, and salt, and blend until smooth and creamy.

3. Add the dill and pulse briefly to incorporate it.

4. Store in a closed container in the refrigerator for up to 2 days.

VARIATION

- Substitute ½ small avocado (about ½ cup chopped) for ½ cup of the cucumber; add more water to adjust the consistency.

SUNFLOWER-SESAME DIP OR DRESSING

SOAK: AT LEAST 4 HOURS ▪ **PREP:** 10 MINUTES   makes about 1 cup dip or 1½ cups dressing GF DF

This is my vegan, soy-free version of "veganaise." It is white, creamy, tangy, slightly bitter, and mustardy as well as rich in good fats, protein, calcium, and iron—perfect for when you're feeling Airy or Earthy.

Aside from topping quick raw salads, Sunflower-Sesame Dressing goes well with Stir-Fried Red and Black Rice (page 154), Kale and Roasted Sweet Potatoes (page 173), Sprouted Mung Salad (page 78), or Black Lentil Soup (page 105). If you are serving it at a party or a family gathering, make extra because people tend to ask for seconds.

¼ cup plus 1 tablespoon white sesame seeds

½ teaspoon black mustard seeds

⅓ cup sunflower seeds, soaked for at least 4 hours or overnight

½ cup water for a dip (or 1 cup for a dressing)

2½ tablespoons fresh lime juice

2½ tablespoons olive oil

1 teaspoon grated fresh ginger

½ teaspoon black salt

¼ teaspoon salt

FOR FIERY DIGESTION: Substitute fennel seeds for the black mustard seeds in Step 1. Substitute more plain salt for the black salt.

1. In a small skillet, dry-toast the sesame seeds and black mustard seeds over low heat while stirring or shaking almost constantly, until the sesame seeds turn slightly golden and the mustard seeds begin to pop. Remove them from the pan to a plate and set aside to cool, then grind to a powder in a spice grinder.

2. Drain and rinse the soaked sunflower seeds.

3. Place all the ingredients in a blender and blend on high speed to a smooth, creamy consistency.

4. To store, keep in a closed container in the refrigerator for up to 3 days. The dressing thickens when refrigerated, so add a little water to thin it as needed.

VARIATION

▪ Pulse in ¼ cup chopped fresh herbs such as basil, parsley, or cilantro in Step 3.

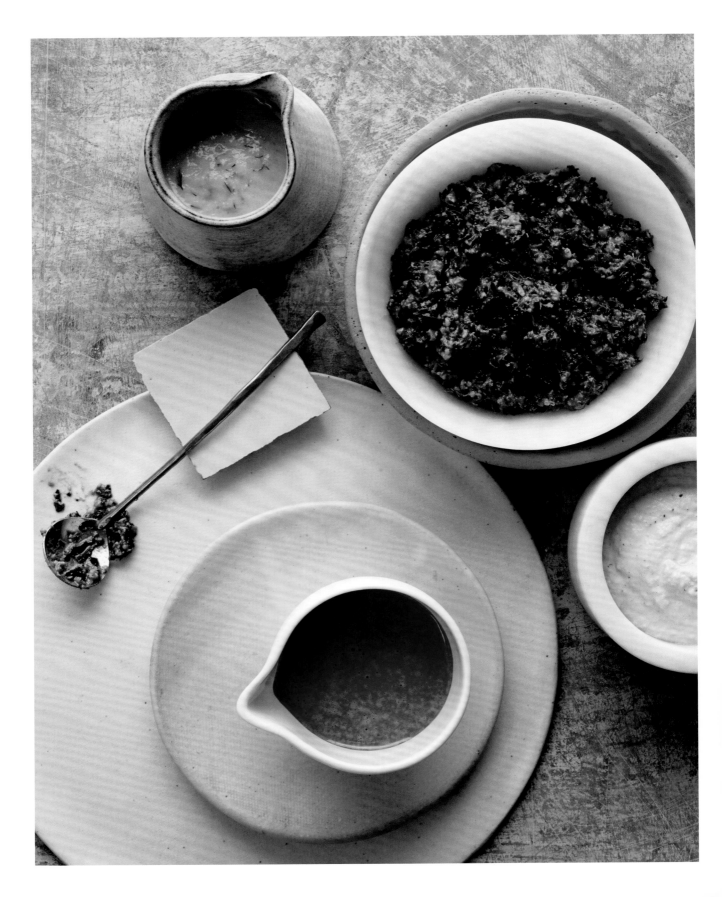

PINK TAHINI DRESSING

PREP: 10 MINUTES

makes ¾ cup GF DF

For a colorful menu, why not use a pink dressing for a change? Reduce the water and salt to create a dip or a spread.

½ teaspoon cumin seeds

½ teaspoon coriander seeds

¼ cup tahini

⅓ cup water

2 tablespoons fresh lime juice

3 tablespoons fresh red beet juice
   (optional; see Note)

¾ teaspoon salt

⅛ teaspoon asafoetida (optional)

1. In a small skillet, dry-toast the cumin seeds and coriander seeds over medium-low heat until the seeds release their aroma and turn a shade darker. Grind to a powder in a spice grinder.

2. Transfer to a blender, add the remaining ingredients, and blend until smooth. Add a little more water to thin the dressing if needed.

3. To store, keep in a closed container in the refrigerator for up to 3 days.

NOTE

- To make the beet juice: Grate a small beet and use your hand or a hand press to squeeze out the juice (use a glove if you don't want to stain your hand). For a white dressing, omit the beet juice.

CLOCKWISE FROM TOP LEFT: Creamy Cucumber Dressing, Kale and Arugula Pesto, Sunflower-Sesame Dip, Pink Tahini Dressing

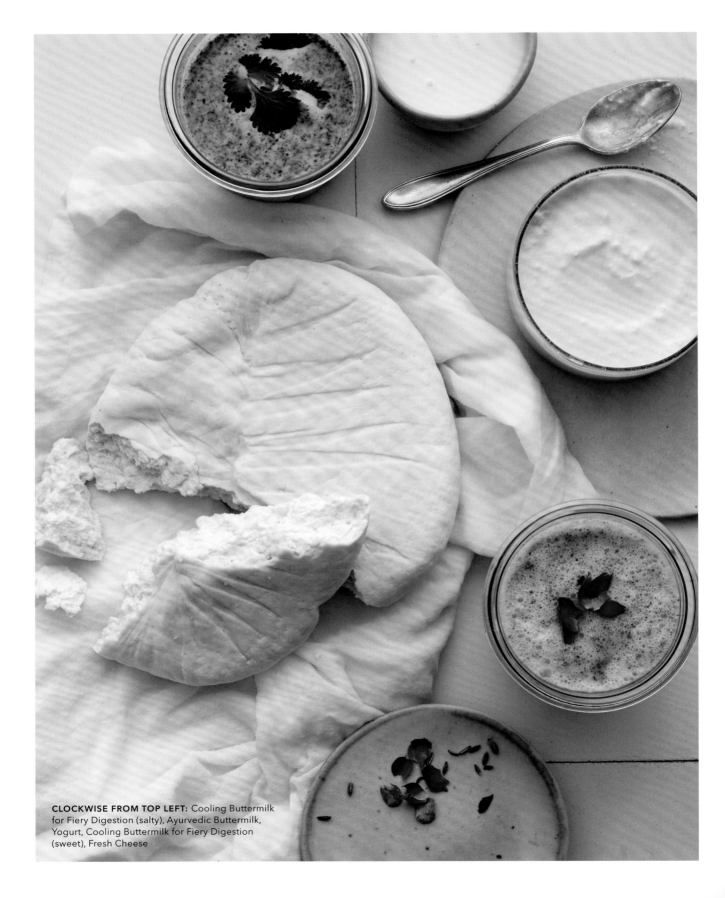

CLOCKWISE FROM TOP LEFT: Cooling Buttermilk for Fiery Digestion (salty), Ayurvedic Buttermilk, Yogurt, Cooling Buttermilk for Fiery Digestion (sweet), Fresh Cheese

THE NEW AYURVEDIC KITCHEN STAPLES

FRESH CHEESE, YOGURT, CULTURED GHEE, BUTTERMILK, ALMOND MILK, AND COCONUT MILK

Freshness is one of the main principles of all healthy cooking. Using canned almond milk, coconut milk, or prepackaged yogurt, cheese, and butter is tempting, but no canned or prepackaged food can provide you with the healing intelligence, benefits, taste, and satisfaction of freshly made staples. Compare the feeling of opening a can to the amusement and pleasure you get every time you squeeze out almond milk or taste your homemade yogurt. There's nothing like it.

In this chapter I want to show you how easy it is to make these basic recipe staples yourself. In our classes I have watched hundreds of people make these recipes for the first time, and they were successful without fail. Preparing staples yourself is empowering and rewarding, something you can teach to your kids and be proud of sharing with your family and friends. I grew up watching my grandmother make yogurt and cheese—it was no big deal, just part of her daily routine. Now every time I make my own dairy products, I think of her and of our ancestors, who knew the art of making staples from scratch. You also can do it yourself.

The staples in this chapter, including almond milk and coconut milk, as well as dairy staples such as fresh cheese (paneer), ghee, and yogurt, are part of many of the book's recipes. To save time preparing those recipes, you may make the staples ahead of time and follow the tips I give on storage.

FRESH CHEESE

Homemade fresh cheese comes in two main forms: soft or pressed. It is the simplest kind of unfermented cheese; it really is the best cheese to eat. The quality and freshness of the milk will determine the quality of the cheese. You must use whole milk; low-fat or skim milk will yield very little or no cheese because the cheese depends on the fat. The higher the fat content of the milk, the richer the cheese.

All fresh cheese is made from curdled milk. Different curdling agents will produce different types of cheese (see chart, below, and Notes, opposite, for ratios). The best curdling agent for creamier, ricotta-like cheese is fresh yogurt or buttermilk; for lower fat and pressed cheese, fresh lime juice works great. You may also use fresh lemon juice or sour whey from a previous batch of curd cheese. Each curdling agent gives a slightly different texture and flavor to the curd—the more acidic the agent, the stiffer the cheese.

Making cheese can be somewhat unpredictable. How long it takes, the quantity produced, and its flavor and texture depend not only on the sourness of the curdling agent but also on the temperature, the kind of pot you use, and the quality of the milk. Do not panic! The more you practice making cheese, the more you will learn to control these variables to suit your preference. Simply follow the basic procedure described below and adjust the details until your cheese is ready. It's easier than you think. Have fun!

Fresh cheese is extremely versatile. It combines well with salads, leafy greens, and vegetables, especially the non-starchy type: summer squash, broccoli, cabbage, cauliflower, and more.

MILK	FRESH LIME JUICE	APPROXIMATE YIELD OF CHEESE
4 cups (1 quart)	2 tablespoons	¾ cup
6 cups (1½ quarts)	3 tablespoons	1⅛ cups
8 cups (2 quarts)	4 tablespoons	1½ cups
10 cups (2½ quarts)	⅓ cup	2 cups
16 cups (1 gallon)	⅓ cup plus 2 tablespoons	3 cups

Take a heavy-based saucepan big enough to contain the milk plus 3 to 4 inches of room for it to foam and boil. Add just enough water to the saucepan to cover its bottom—this magic trick will protect the pot from getting crusty and it will ease your cleaning afterward. Then pour the milk in and bring to a boil over medium heat (cooking it over high heat can cause the milk to scorch and stick).

The moment the milk starts to boil, reduce the heat to low and add the lime juice or other curdling agent (see note about curdling with yogurt or buttermilk). Stir gently until the milk curdles. This is what you are looking for: the milk has to transform into clumpy curds and yellowish whey. If the gently boiling liquid still looks milky white, it has not fully curdled yet; add more lime juice and stir until the whey clears. Once the curds separate from the whey, turn off the heat immediately; this is important because leaving the heat on will make the cheese tough or crumbly.

There are two ways to strain, depending on what form of cheese you need:

To make soft crumbled cheese: Pour or scoop the curds into a mesh strainer (no cheesecloth needed) and let them drain until the desired texture.

To make pressed cheese (aka paneer) for cutting into cubes or grating: Pour or scoop the curds into a colander or mesh strainer lined with cheesecloth, gather the corners of the cloth, making sure that the cheese is tightly enclosed, and hold the bag under lukewarm water for 5 to 10 seconds

(be careful not to burn yourself—the curds will be very hot). Then gently twist the cloth to squeeze out the excess whey; place on a smooth flat surface and press the bundled curds with something heavy like a pan or pot. There are several ways to press the cheese; it depends on what you have available. When I'm pressing a bigger amount of cheese in my kitchen, I usually insert the curd bundle between two cutting boards and then place a cast-iron pan on top. For a smaller amount, you may place the bundled curds in a colander and press it with a full bowl of water or another heavy weight; a tofu press works perfectly as well. Press until the cheese is firm enough to hold itself together but is still soft and spongy. Pressing 1 to 2 cups of cheese with a cast-iron pan should not take more than 20 minutes. Do not leave the cheese pressed for too long because then it will become hard to eat and digest. Unwrap your homemade cheese and use as directed in a recipe.

NOTES

- If you would like to use yogurt or buttermilk as curdling agents in Step 2, use these proportions: ½ cup plain yogurt or ⅔ cup plain buttermilk for every 4 cups milk.

- Whey is nutritious, but it is best to avoid consuming it because it is very acidic and rather difficult to digest.

- It is best to consume fresh cheese right away, but you may also seal it in a bag or a closed container and refrigerate it for up to 3 days.

The Healing Benefits of Fresh Cheese

Fresh cheese is sweet, heavy to digest, and aphrodisiac. Its fatty properties are superb for the Airy and the Fiery; Earthy types need it in less quantity, less frequently, and with extra servings of pungent spices.

Fresh cheese is rich in animal protein, calcium, vitamin B12, and omega fatty acids, and is an important ingredient in a vegetarian diet. Since it is a heavy food, you can try these tips to make it easier to digest:

- Eat it freshly made, while the protein molecules are not fully bound and hardened.

- Eat it at lunchtime, when digestion is strongest.

- Add digestive spices such as black pepper, cardamom (black or green), green chiles, and ginger.

- Avoid combining it in a dish or a meal with contradictory foods such as fruit (see "Learning to Mix and Match for Delicious, Digestible Meals"; page 36).

- Choose cow's or goat's milk cheeses. Sheep's dairy aggravates almost every digestive system, and buffalo dairy is very heavy (recommended only for sleeplessness and excessive hunger pangs).

Fresh vs. Fermented Cheeses

In Ayurveda, we rank foods in terms of freshness and digestion: the less fresh and harder to digest an ingredient is, the less healthy it is. Aged for months or even years, fermented cheeses are very acidic and lower the body's pH, creating a favorable environment for inflammation and unwanted bacteria or fungi to thrive. They are much heavier to digest and therefore can easily block our microcirculatory channels.

Ayurvedic cheeses are always fresh. They are not ripened with bacteria, rennet, or enzymes or washed with alcohol such as brandy or beer. Their aroma is sweet and heavenly, not stinky like a pair of dirty socks. They are delightful, light, and when properly combined with other foods will not cause mucus or blockages. The following list ranks cheese in terms of digestibility, with fresh homemade cheese the most easily digested (and the only cheese I fully recommend using) and aged and hard cheeses the most difficult to digest.

1. Fresh homemade cheese (paneer)

2. Organic unripened soft cheese: cottage cheese, ricotta, fresh mozzarella, goat cheese

3. Soft/rind-ripened cheeses: Brie, Camembert

4. Semisoft cheeses that are only aged for up to a month: fresh feta, mozzarella

5. Aged and hard cheeses: cheddar, Parmesan, blue cheese, dry Monterey Jack

YOGURT

Having grown up in Bulgaria, known for its exceptional yogurt, I am very attached to yogurt's taste, probiotic strength, and consistency—that's why I like to make it myself.

A good-quality yogurt is a trusted source of healing friendly bacteria, protein, calcium, essential digestive enzymes, and vitamin B12. For a person with good digestion, the bio-availability of these nutrients is about 80 percent; in other words, small amounts of yogurt consumed regularly will deliver these essential nutrients.

In my studies of Ayurveda, I've learned that there are three types of yogurt, based on taste: sweet, sour, and very sour. The best quality yogurt is sweet with a slight sour and astringent aftertaste. This yogurt carries the many healing benefits listed below. Sour yogurt increases acidity and can be very aggravating for the Fiery and the Earthy.

Creamy throughout with a bliss-producing layer of cream on top, homemade yogurt is far superior to its commercial counterparts, which are often tangy or slimy and packed with unnecessary stabilizers or preservatives such as gelatin, carrageenan, cellulose, pectin, or cornstarch.

Many variables can affect the outcome of your yogurt, including timing, temperature, humidity, drafts, and the quality of milk. Don't be discouraged if you don't get a firm set yogurt the first time. Try again; it's worth the effort. For gourmet and therapeutic results, use the best quality milk (see the "Milk Glossary" on page 243) and a thermometer with a temperature range of 0 to 220°F, which you can find at kitchenware stores, restaurant supplies stores, and online. See Sources (page 250) for where to find a good-quality yogurt starter.

1 quart whole unhomogenized milk
¼ cup plain, full-fat yogurt

HEATING THE MILK
Slowly heat the milk in a heavy 3-quart pan to 180 to 190°F and keep it at this temperature for 15 minutes, stirring occasionally. This will make the yogurt sweeter, thicker, and creamier.

COOLING THE MILK
Set aside ½ cup milk in a bowl and let it cool to room temperature. Whisk in the yogurt (your starter) to a creamy consistency.

Let the rest of the milk cool to 115°F. The longer the milk cools, the thicker and tastier the finished product will be. If you are pressed for time, do a quick cool by placing the milk pan in a kitchen sink or a bowl half-full of cold water (be careful not to splash water in the milk). You may also stir the milk to accelerate the cooling.

Use a thermometer to ensure proper temperature. A temperature of 110 to 115°F is important so that the bacteria will thrive and the yogurt will set properly.

ADDING THE STARTER
Gently stir the yogurt starter mixture into the milk and mix thoroughly. Now the milk temperature should be near 108 to 112°F, which is ideal for starting yogurt. Leave the

milk in a covered pot or bowl or transfer it to a jar or another container with a lid.

INCUBATING THE YOGURT

Now it's time for the friendly bacteria to grow and transform the milk into yogurt. The key is to keep it warm (85 to 110°F) for 5 to 6 hours. There are many ways to do that:

- Wrap the container in a clean towel or blanket and keep it in a warm spot.

- Place the container in a food dehydrator at 110°F.

- Keep it near a heater.

- Use a yogurt maker: follow the manufacturer's instructions for incubation.

- Put it in a gas oven: heat to 200°F for 1 to 2 minutes, turn it off, and place the container on the top shelf in the back. Do not put yogurt in an oven above 120°F.

- Put it in an electric oven: heat to 200°F for 1 to 2 minutes and turn it off. Wrap the container in a towel and place on any shelf. Leave the oven light on. Do not put yogurt in an oven above 120°F.

Be careful, because if the environment is too hot, the yogurt will sour before it sets and become very watery.

HOW DO YOU KNOW WHEN IT'S YOGURT?

Check the yogurt after 5 to 6 hours. If you are incubating overnight, stop the process as soon as you get up in the morning.

Yogurt is ready when it is thick and firm, with a custard-like appearance that separates from the edge of the container. If longer incubation is needed, check every 30 minutes.

REFRIGERATION AND STORAGE

It is best to refrigerate the yogurt and leave it undisturbed for several hours until thoroughly chilled. This will firm it up and preserve its sweetness. As it is 100 percent natural, without any stabilizers or preservatives, the yogurt will release whey. This whey is good stuff—unlike whey from fresh cheese, yogurt whey is less acidic and rich in friendly bacteria; you can either mix it in or pour it into a cup and drink it as a probiotic. I like to use a teaspoon of the yogurt whey for facial masks to enrich my skin with friendly bacteria.

To benefit from the fresh yogurt's sweet taste and strongest bacteria, it is best to use it within 5 days. As the yogurt ages, its probiotic properties will weaken and it will become more sour.

NOTES

- Do not heat the milk in a microwave oven!

- If you do not have a thermometer and want to determine whether the milk is cool enough to add the starter, make your pinky a thermometer: if you can dip it in the cooling milk and hold for ten seconds, the temperature is about right.

- My favorite vessel for incubating yogurt is a non-glazed clay pot.

- If you make yogurt with a powdered starter, follow the product directions.

- If you're making yogurt with raw milk, when you heat the milk, bring it to a full boil, then reduce the heat and simmer for 15 minutes.

- For the next batch of homemade yogurt, reserve the starter in a small jar and label it.

- If you make yogurt from goat's milk, it may be more liquidy because goat's milk's protein-to-fat ratio is different from that of cow's milk.

The Healing Benefits of Yogurt

The ancients describe yogurt as one of the most beneficial substances on earth. Here are some of its healing benefits (again, this describes the best quality yogurt):

- Cleanses the taste buds and enhances our ability to taste food

- Stimulates digestion (a great source of digestive enzymes)

- Supports absorption of nutrients

- Lubricates the body's channels

- Increases stamina

- Is a good body-builder

- Is a diuretic

Yogurt Do's and Don'ts

Do's with Yogurt

- When mixing into cooked grains, vegetables, or soups, gradually stir in the yogurt after turning off the heat; otherwise it will break up and curdle.

- For most people, the best time of day to eat yogurt is between 10 a.m. and 2 p.m., when digestion is strongest.

- Sprinkle yogurt with a pinch of nutmeg or cinnamon to aid digestion.

Don'ts with Yogurt

- Do not mix yogurt (in a dish or a meal) with fruit, nightshades, leafy greens, or milk—these combinations put a heavy load on your digestive fire and may lead to imbalances.

- Avoid eating yogurt at night—it might be too much for your digestion.

- Discard any partially fermented yogurt (when it has the signs of fermentation but it's still quite liquid). This substance will aggravate everyone's physiology. It might break your heart to waste it, but better that than increased toxins in your body.

- Refrain from eating old yogurt. It will not only increase acidity but may also cause flatulence, inflammation, water retention, or problems with urination.

CULTURED GHEE

makes about 20 ounces

If I had to choose one staple I couldn't go without, that would be ghee. It is the magical golden substance that makes everything cook well and taste better. Ghee has been glorified throughout the Vedas, used through centuries in cooking and yogic rituals, and included in numerous Ayurvedic remedies. I am so glad that more and more nutritionists and naturopaths today value ghee's nurturing properties and recommend it as an essential component of a healthy diet.

Ghee is the deeply nourishing core essence of milk. It has all the micronutrients and antioxidants of butter but without butter's water, milk protein (casein), and lactose. I've met many lactose-intolerant people who do not react to ghee. In fact, cultured ghee helped them repair their gut damage.

There are two types of ghee, depending on how its starting ingredient, butter, is derived: 1) from sweet cream, and 2) from cultured cream. The first type I call "regular" ghee—it is higher in cholesterol and it increases body fat; it is the ghee widely sold and used today. The second type, known as "cultured" or "probiotic" ghee, decreases bad cholesterol and regulates fat metabolism; it is really the best ghee to cook with, but it is harder to find. What distinguishes cultured ghee from even organic store-bought products is the culturing of cream as the first step. The culture infuses the cream or butter with beneficial bacteria, making it easier to digest and thus promoting overall health.

The subtlest requirement for ghee making is a proper environment because ghee is highly absorbent, both physically and energetically. Make sure your "ghee kitchen" is a clean and peaceful space; you may even play a continuous recording of sacred music or chants. Make ghee when you feel happy and settled, free from negative thoughts. Some healers recommend making therapeutic ghee during a waxing moon or a few hours before the full moon, when nurturing energy in the environment is on the rise.

In this recipe, I want to share the traditional secrets for making cultured ghee that I have learned from one of my Ayurvedic teachers, Vaidya R. K. Mishra. The process of churning your own butter and transforming it into "liquid gold" is not only alchemical; it is truly magical. Note that there are so many ways you can cut corners when making ghee, but if you want the best, curative product, make it without compromise. If you are unable to make your own cultured butter, you can follow my "Quick Ghee Making" guidelines on page 211 using store-bought cultured butter. Making ghee may seem intimidating at first, but with practice it becomes easy and enjoyable. Keep in mind that the larger the quantity, the longer the cooking time.

CLOCKWISE FROM TOP LEFT: fresh butter, cultured cream, hot ghee, solidified ghee

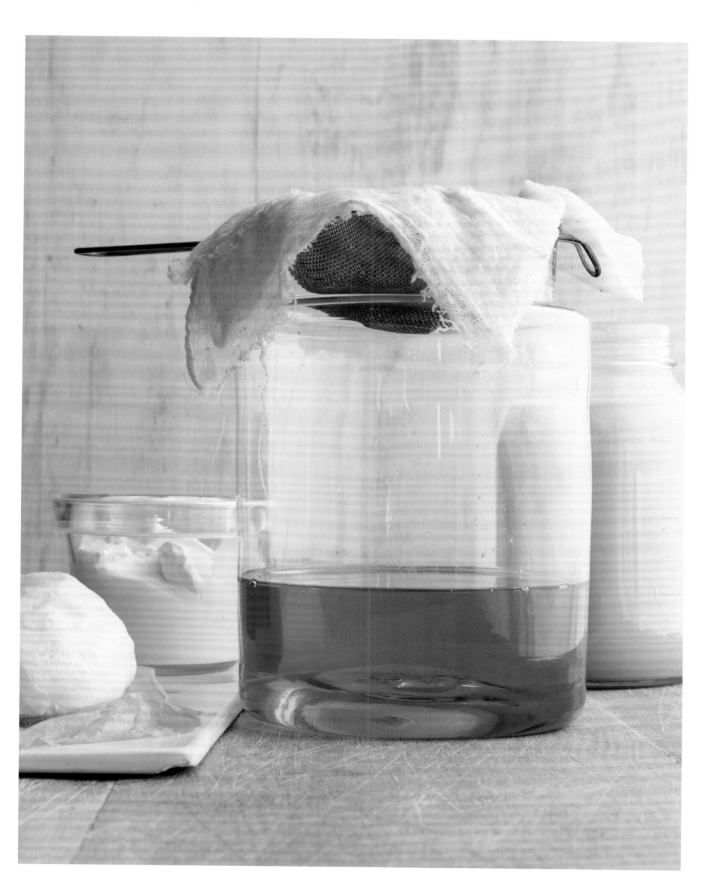

4 pints raw or pasteurized organic, grass-fed heavy whipping cream (do not use ultrapasteurized)

1 cup plain, full-fat organic yogurt or 2 teaspoons Natren yogurt starter (see Sources, page 250)

UTENSILS AND EQUIPMENT

Food processor fitted with the "S" blade or standing mixer set with the wire beaters (a blender does not work well for butter churning)

Sieve

2 mixing bowls

Rubber scraper

Heavy 3- or 4-quart pan that heats evenly on all sides

Wooden cooking spoon

Dry cheesecloth or flour-sack towel

Dry sieve and a bowl

Jars for storing

CULTURING THE CREAM

Follow the instructions for making yogurt (page 205), but substitute heavy whipping cream for the whole milk. Let the cultured cream chill completely. You will be tempted to stop there and indulge in the delicious, custard-like cream-yogurt—taste a teaspoon as an educational experience, but keep going!

CHURNING CULTURED CREAM INTO BUTTER

The quantity of cultured cream you churn at a time depends on the volume capacity of the appliance you're using. Whether churning with a food processor, a standing mixer, or another butter churner, fill it with cream-yogurt halfway and turn it onto one of the highest speeds. Within a minute (or

a couple of minutes, depending on the volume), the cream-yogurt will transform into thick whipped cream that will gradually loosen up and become sloshy. At this point, turn to the lowest speed (if that's an option). As it keeps churning and looks more and more buttery, gradually lower the speed to the lowest setting, when the cream breaks and you hear a splashing sound. Now you have produced two marvelous products: the fresh butter and buttermilk. When they have fully separated and the butter clusters into a ball, turn off the churning device.

Transfer the churned butter to a sieve over a mixing bowl. Press the butter between your hands to press and squeeze out the buttermilk as much as possible. You may be tempted to slather some gleaming butter on toast right now, yes? Be patient; you're not done yet.

COOKING BUTTER INTO GHEE

Place the fresh butter in a 3- to 4-quart heavy pot; turn on the burner to the lowest possible setting. Stir occasionally as the butter melts and starts to bubble. Notice how the three components of butter begin to separate: water will be on the bottom, butterfat will take up most of the pot, and milk fat solids will mostly rise to the top. As the temperature rises to 200°F, the separation will become more and more distinct; the water will bubble up, maybe with a few eruptions. Many cooks skim the foam on top to speed up their ghee making—that's not the traditional way; it's best to let the foam disappear naturally.

Stir the pot occasionally in order to avoid sediment burning and to help the water evaporate. Thermodynamic physicists will explain why the butter oil resists serious heating until the water is gone. For us cooks, we're happy as long as the butter is cooking without burning.

When the solids have more or less settled to the bottom (as opposed to floating around), stop stirring from the bottom up. Let the milk fat solids rest at the bottom. Because the water is reduced, the temperature rises faster and the butterfat begins to lose its cloudiness; the large bubbles you saw earlier have turned into thin foam.

The ghee is ready when the butter oil is clear, amber in color, and the solids you see on the bottom of the pan are consistent golden brown. You should be able to clearly see the bottom of the pan. Light tan or blackish solids are not good signs. If the solids are mostly tan, keep the ghee in the refrigerator between uses. If the solids have become black, you've scorched the ghee and all its healing properties—remorsefully, you will have to discard it.

STRAINING THE GHEE
Fold the cheesecloth into 8 layers (2 layers if you're using a flour-sack towel) and place it in a strainer atop a mixing bowl. From now on, all utensils the ghee comes in contact with must be completely dry, as moisture will spoil the ghee. Carefully pour or ladle the hot ghee through the cheesecloth. You want to do this quickly. If the temperature drops below 200°F, the fatty nutrients so important to the ghee begin to crystalize. Discard the strained solids. To clean and reuse the cheesecloth, soak it in boiling hot water with soap; hand-wash while the soapy water is still warm.

Let the ghee cool for a few minutes, allowing for any air molecules to dissipate. Pour the ghee into glass jars. Put the lids on only when the jars have cooled to room temperature in order to avoid condensation falling in the ghee. Transfer the closed jars to the refrigerator—this will prevent the formation of layers. Once the ghee has solidified, transfer the jars to a dry and dark space such as a cabinet.

STORING THE GHEE
Ghee has a long shelf life at room temperature, generally months, but it's best to keep the unused jars refrigerated and the jar you're currently cooking with in the cabinet. Store it in the dark between meals and protect it from even a drop of moisture.

QUICK GHEE MAKING
I am aware that most cooks do not have the time, patience, or motivation to churn their own butter from cultured cream. Quick Ghee is the next best option, but unfortunately it will not grant you the benefit of fresh buttermilk as a by-product. Purchase organic, grass-fed, unsalted *cultured butter* (Organic Valley's is excellent) and follow the above instructions for cooking butter into ghee. You can make ghee with regular sweet cream butter, but it will be lacking the probiotic goodness and it will be higher in cholesterol. Whatever butter you use, make sure it is unsalted and organic, ideally grass-fed.

The Healing Benefits of Cultured Ghee

Here's what I have learned from the ancient Ayurvedic texts about ghee:

- Enhances digestive fire while having a cooling and alkalizing effect on the whole body

- Calms and rejuvenates the eyes

- Promotes longevity

- Binds fat-soluble toxins

- Cools and lubricates the stomach wall

- Pacifies the Airy and the Fiery

- Enhances complexion and glow of the face and body

- Increases physical and mental stamina

- Supports the brain's functions of learning, retention, and recall

And here are some additional findings from modern research:

- Gives satiation

- Provides sustaining energy

- Supports healthy hormone production

- Enhances mineral absorption

- Helps the delivery and absorption of fat-soluble vitamins A, D, E, and K

- Produces healthy bile by supporting the liver

- Maintains anti-inflammatory processes and supports the body's healing intelligence

General Guidelines for Cooking with Ghee

- Ghee's smoke point is 485°F and it is an ideal base oil for boiling, sautéing, baking, roasting, and pan-frying (even deep-frying, although I don't recommend it).

- Melt the ghee on medium-low heat to fry spices, flatbreads, or omelets or to sauté vegetables. Protect it from smoking and burning, as burned ghee is very unhealthy and should be discarded.

- Never reuse ghee (or any oil!) left after cooking. Once the ghee is heated beyond its smoke point, it oxidizes and its fats begin to decompose, forming toxic compounds.

- Anyone with heart, liver, or kidney imbalance should consult a medical professional before using ghee.

- Discard rancid ghee (whitish in color).

- Yes, you may spread it on hot toast!

AYURVEDIC BUTTERMILK

PREP: 2 MINUTES makes 1 cup

More than five thousand years ago the ancients considered buttermilk "nectar on earth," and it is still so today. It is a marvelous elixir, rich in highly intelligent bacteria, ideally suited to making your digestive system healthy. "Health begins in the gut," Hippocrates wisely noted. The optimal digestive functions of absorption, assimilation, and elimination depend on the proper quality and quantity of friendly flora in the gut. How amazing it is that unassuming buttermilk can give that to us!

A lot of people nowadays take probiotic capsules, and they can be very helpful for a few months. But do not let your system depend on them on an ongoing basis. Once the probiotic supplements have won the battle over unfriendly bacteria (and even candida!), the battlefield of your gut is clear to refertilize it and grow an abundance of beneficial flora in a more natural way—by regularly consuming best-quality yogurt, buttermilk, and other cultured foods.

Let us welcome the probiotic wonderment of buttermilk in our diet and invite its little friendly constituents to be happy and thrive in the fields of our digestive system. All you need is ½ to 1 cup of buttermilk daily or even three to four times a week. As with yogurt, the best time to enjoy buttermilk is midday—during or right after lunch.

There are two main ways to produce homemade buttermilk: 1) By churning cultured cream into butter (see Cultured Ghee, page 208)—the liquid that separates from the butter is called buttermilk 2) By following the recipe below—that's faster.

I use buttermilk in several recipes in this book—mostly for baking and making digestive beverages.

¼ cup plain, full-fat yogurt (ideally
    homemade)
¾ cup spring or filtered water

Blend the yogurt and water until a buttery froth forms on the surface (any kind of blender will work). Skim and discard the froth—this lowers the fat in the buttermilk and makes it lighter. Blending is important, as it infuses the buttermilk with more Fiery energy, thus enhancing its digestive powers. Your staple buttermilk is ready to use in recipes!

The Healing Benefits of Buttermilk

These benefits described by the ancients must be true today too:

- Supports absorption of nutrients

- Restores healthy appetite

- Balances fat metabolism and cholesterol

- Supports weight reduction

- Restores the intelligence of the colon

- Alleviates hemorrhoids

- Improves circulation

- Is good for the spleen

DIGESTIVE BUTTERMILKS

There are many variations of digestive buttermilk recipes; here are a few quick ones. The preparation method is the same, but you can vary ingredients depending on your digestion. Always serve digestive buttermilk at room temperature. All the recipes below make one serving.

STRENGTHENING BUTTERMILK FOR AIRY DIGESTION

PREP: 5 MINUTES   makes 1 cup

Excellent for when you're experiencing fluctuating digestive fire.

¼ teaspoon Digestive Masala (page 223)
⅛ teaspoon plain salt or black salt
1 cup Ayurvedic Buttermilk (page 213)

Gently dry-toast the masala in a small skillet over low heat until it darkens a shade and releases its aroma. Pulse in a blender with the salt and buttermilk.

COOLING BUTTERMILK FOR FIERY DIGESTION

PREP: 5 MINUTES   makes 1 cup

Ideal for acidic digestion or when you feel excessive hunger or heat.

SWEET
½ teaspoon fennel seeds
1 dried rosebud or ½ teaspoon rose petals
2 teaspoons coconut palm sugar or raw cane sugar, or to taste
½ teaspoon rose water
1 cup Ayurvedic Buttermilk (page 213)

Dry-toast the fennel seeds and rosebud in a small skillet over low heat until they darken a shade and release their aroma. Grind to a powder in a spice grinder. Pulse in a blender with the sugar, rose water, and buttermilk.

SALTY
¼ teaspoon cumin seeds
1 tablespoon chopped cilantro leaves
⅛ teaspoon salt
1 cup Ayurvedic Buttermilk (page 213)

Dry-toast the cumin seeds in a small skillet over low heat until they darken a shade and release their aroma. Grind to a powder in a spice grinder. Pulse in a blender with the cilantro, salt, and buttermilk.

ENERGIZING BUTTERMILK FOR EARTHY DIGESTION

PREP: 5 MINUTES makes 1 cup

Slightly sour yogurt is preferred for this recipe, but sweet will also do. Yogurt is generally too heavy and clogging for the Earthy; this recipe is one of the best ways to benefit from the friendly bacteria of yogurt without feeling heavy.

⅛ teaspoon black peppercorns
¼ teaspoon cumin seeds
⅛ teaspoon fenugreek seeds
⅛ teaspoon powdered ginger
1 cup Ayurvedic Buttermilk (page 213)

Dry-toast the black peppercorns, cumin seeds, and fenugreek seeds in a small skillet over low heat until they darken a shade and release their aroma. Grind to a powder in a spice grinder. Pulse in a blender with the ginger and buttermilk.

The Difference Between Ayurvedic Buttermilk and Lassi

Ayurvedic buttermilk (aka *takra* in Sanskrit and Hindi) and lassi are slightly different: buttermilk is made according to the recipe on page 213, by blending it and removing the fatty froth, which makes it almost fat-free and easy to digest.

Lassi uses the same blended ingredients of the buttermilk recipe (and sometimes more yogurt and less water), but without removing the fatty froth. SV Ayurveda recommends drinking lassi only when you have really strong hunger; otherwise, choose buttermilk. Traditional Ayurvedic lassi by far excels the beverages sold by the same name in Indian restaurants!

Buttermilk and lassi are not the same as kefir, which contains different cultures and is more heavy and sour (and thus heating). Nowadays most of us have trouble digesting acidic foods, so be careful with store-bought kefir. Try fresh homemade kefir and see how your stomach responds.

ALMOND MILK

Making almond milk is quick and uncomplicated. It takes less time to make it at home than to go to the store and buy it. If you have been drinking boxed almond milk, you'll taste a big difference with your fresh, homemade version. I guarantee you that after milking your almonds a couple of times, making your own almond milk will become second nature, and you will never need to look at the recipe again.

1 cup raw almonds (ideally unpasteurized)
3 cups spring or filtered water
Small pinch of salt (optional)

Place the almonds in a bowl, jar, or other container, rinse them, and cover with cold spring or filtered water, making sure there is at least 2 inches of water above the almonds. Refrigerate and soak for 8 to 12 hours. Refrigerating protects the almonds from fermenting; you may keep soaking the almonds in the fridge for longer than 12 hours, up to 5 days; just make sure to change the water every day.

Drain the nuts and rinse them well. (Peeling the almonds at this point is ideal but optional.) Place them in a blender with the filtered water and salt, if using (the salt brings out the almond flavor). Blend on high speed until the nuts are completely broken down; the timing depends on the blender, but it shouldn't take more than a minute.

Place a nut milk bag over a bowl, pour the mixture through a corner of the bag (layered cheesecloth also works, but it's harder to clean), and squeeze out as much of the milk as possible. Now you have delicious fresh almond milk to enjoy on its own or use for other recipes.

To store your almond milk, pour it into a jar or an airtight container and refrigerate for up to 3 days. Shake well before using.

NOTES

▪ Wondering what to do with the almond pulp? The remaining almond pulp is good stuff; do not discard it. Be creative how to use it: with your oatmeal, in a salad or dressing, for cookies, or Sesame Honey Balls (page 86), for example. If you don't need it immediately, here are some ways to store it:

▪ Cover and refrigerate for up to 2 days

▪ Freeze for up to a month

▪ Dehydrate right away at 95°F until completely dry and store in a closed container. It will keep on a shelf for a long time; use it to make sprouted almond meal or almond flour.

The Healing Benefits of Almonds

Ayurveda describes almonds as sweet, heating, and hard to digest. Soaking the almonds makes them easier to digest and balancing for the Airy, Fiery, and Earthy. Almonds nourish the brain, support the male reproductive system, and are an excellent tonic for restoring energy. Soaked almonds are great during pregnancy.

COCONUT MILK

makes about 1½ cups coconut milk per young coconut
(yield varies depending on how meaty your coconut is)

In my earlier years of cooking, I never bought coconuts from the grocery store because I didn't know how to handle them. Opening a can of coconut milk seemed so much easier. But once I tasted freshly made coconut milk, I could not believe the difference—its bursting sweet aroma filled the room, and its white creaminess emanated vitality. I was converted. Not only does fresh coconut milk taste better, but all its vitamins and minerals are intact—something canned coconut milk lacks.

You can make coconut milk from mature (brown hard shell) coconuts, but my preference is to use young (Thai), green-skinned coconuts because of their milk's creamier consistency and stronger flavor.

The basic method is this: open the coconut, drain the water, scoop out the meat, and blend it with water. This process is a bit tricky because each coconut is different and you never know how much coconut meat you will get until you open it. That's why I usually buy at least one extra coconut, just in case the others are a bit short on meat.

1 young coconut

Enough spring or filtered water to blend to desired consistency (1 to 2 cups)

OPENING THE COCONUT

Tilt the coconut to one side (with the pointed tip up), and using a sharp knife, shave the top husk, exposing the inner shell.

With the square corner of the knife's blade (by the hilt), pierce the exposed coconut shell and begin tapping and going around in a circle—almost like opening a can—until you can open the "lid." Pour the coconut water through a strainer into a bowl. Save the water and drink it as soon as you can! It is the best electrolyte drink on earth. Gently scoop the coconut meat out with a metal spoon or a scooper. Clean off any small bits of brown fibrous skin or coconut shell.

MAKING THE COCONUT MILK

Blend the coconut "meat" with 1 cup spring or filtered water until smooth. Check the consistency; if it's too thick, add more water. Your coconut milk is now ready to use in recipes.

Coconut milk will stay fresh for up to 3 days refrigerated in an airtight container.

NOTES

- Make sure the coconut is not moldy and its water does not taste sour.

- Do not cook with coconut water or coconut milk made with coconut water—it turns sour and unhealthy.

- To learn more about the healing benefits of coconut, see Coconut and Papaya Smoothie on page 127.

SPICE BLENDS

On pages 227 to 233 I discuss the importance of cooking with spices. Here are a few spice blends, aka masalas (*masala* is the Hindi word for "spice blend") I use in the recipes throughout the book. You can, of course, incorporate these masalas into many other recipes. The spice blends below are designed for specific digestion, and they also can come in handy when you're speed cooking and don't want to niggle about which single spices to throw in the pot. Plus any of the masalas below make inexpensive, exclusive gifts!

Precooked Spice Blends

Because all the ingredients in the following two recipes are pre-toasted, these precooked blends are added to recipes in the last five minutes of cooking.

FAT-BURNING MASALA

PREP: 10 MINUTES   makes a little more than 1 tablespoon

Fenugreek is quite effective in digesting protein, burning fat, and lowering blood sugar. The bitter seeds become more palatable when dry-toasted and balanced with their antidote, coriander. This masala is suitable for when you're feeling Earthy and for cooking recipes with fresh cheese and starchy vegetables.

4 teaspoons coriander seeds
1 teaspoon fenugreek seeds

Following the technique in the Superspice Masala (page 219), dry-toast the coriander seeds until they darken to golden brown and release their aroma, then dry-toast the fenugreek seeds until they become dark brown (milk chocolate–like in color).

Let the toasted spices cool down; transfer them to an electric grinder or spice mill and grind to a fine powder. Store in an airtight jar away from light.

SUPERSPICE MASALA

PREP: 15 MINUTES

On page 229 I will introduce you to the four superspices, and this masala is a good way to combine them and cook with them. With its mild yellowish color and flavor, it is superb for gently incorporating more spices into your food. If you've never cooked or eaten with these four spices before, start by adding a pinch or two of this masala with each meal. Gradually increase to ½ teaspoon per person per meal. I like to take a small stash of the Superspice Masala when I travel and cannot cook for myself—I sprinkle a couple of pinches of it as a digestive aid on whatever savory food I eat. This blend goes well with any salty dish, such as soups, grains, vegetables, salads, protein, khichari, and buttermilk. If you are a kitchen adventurist, go ahead and blend ½ teaspoon in your vegetable smoothie.

2 tablespoons coriander seeds
2 tablespoons fennel seeds
1 teaspoon cumin seeds
1 teaspoon ground turmeric

Separately dry-toast each spice in a heavy skillet (cast iron works well). The key is to keep the pan on low heat and to stir or shake almost constantly—this will toast the little seeds evenly without burning them. If you burn a spice, discard it and start again.

Start with the coriander seeds because they take longer to toast. The seeds will begin to darken and release their aroma; they are done when they darken to a golden brown color—this could take up to 5 minutes. Immediately transfer the toasted coriander to a dry bowl; repeat the same technique with the fennel seeds, and then with the cumin seeds. Enjoy the aromatherapy as you toast!

Before you proceed with turmeric, turn off the heat and let the pan cool for a minute. Turmeric is a very fine powder that can burn within seconds, so you need to toast it at even lower heat. Add the turmeric to the slightly cooled pan and stir constantly. Within seconds, it will turn deep orange—this is when it's done. Transfer immediately to the bowl of toasted spices. If the turmeric became brown, you have burned it and all of its great properties—just discard it and start again.

Let the toasted spices cool down; transfer them to an electric grinder or spice mill and grind to a fine powder. Store in an airtight jar away from light.

NOTES

- You may omit the dry-toasting steps and simply grind all the spices together in their raw form. Add this raw version of Superspice Masala at the beginning of cooking and let the spices simmer with your food for at least 10 to 15 minutes. This raw blend won't be suitable for just sprinkling on food; you have to cook with it.

- Do not make tea out of this blend.

Raw Spice Blends

The following masala recipes are all prepared by the same method of grinding the raw spices in a spice grinder.

There are two main ways to use the following spice blends:

- Add at the beginning of cooking.

- Add at the end of cooking: For 2 to 4 servings, heat 1 tablespoon ghee or oil over low heat and toast 1 teaspoon masala for 5 to 10 seconds, until the spices release their aroma. Immediately remove from the heat (to prevent burning) and drizzle over cooked rice or vegetables. Cover right away to let the flavors steep.

SWEET MASALA

PREP: 3 MINUTES   makes about ¼ cup

The aroma of this spice blend is most charming—you'll probably find yourself opening its jar once in a while just to smell it. The fragrant yet not overpowering ingredients are excellent for breaking down carbs, sugars, and milk. Use this heavenly masala as the "secret ingredient" for sweet dishes such as cakes, muffins, cookies, smoothies, and oatmeal.

1 tablespoon fennel seeds

1 tablespoon coriander seeds

1 tablespoon dried rose petals or buds

1½ teaspoons cinnamon granules or crushed cinnamon bark

¾ teaspoon cardamom seeds (not pods!)

¾ teaspoon vanilla extract powder

Place all the ingredients in an electric grinder or spice mill and grind to a fine powder. Store in an airtight jar away from light.

NOTE

- If you want to add Sweet Masala to a cake or muffin recipe that does not call for it, use 1 teaspoon of the blend for every 2 cups of flour; or for milk, boil ½ teaspoon of the blend with 1 cup of milk for 5 minutes.

ENERGIZING MASALA

PREP: 5 MINUTES

makes 3 tablespoons

This spice blend stirs up slow digestion and lazy fat metabolism without overheating the liver. It is ideal for weight reduction diets, when you're feeling Earthy, or when you want to shake off winter sluggishness. However, this heating masala is not recommended when you feel Fiery.

1 tablespoon coriander seeds

1 teaspoon fenugreek seeds

1 teaspoon cumin seeds

1 teaspoon ajwain seeds

½ teaspoon powdered ginger

½ teaspoon ground turmeric

¼ teaspoon black peppercorns

¼ teaspoon cinnamon granules or crushed cinnamon bark

¼ teaspoon black cardamom seeds (from 1 or 2 pods)

¼ teaspoon salt

Place all the ingredients in an electric grinder or spice mill and grind to a fine powder. Store in an airtight jar away from light.

COOLING MASALA

PREP: 3 MINUTES

makes about ½ cup

This spice blend is very balancing for when you're feeling Fiery and during hot weather. Add it at the beginning of cooking soups, grains, leafy greens, or vegetables.

3 tablespoons coriander seeds

3 tablespoons fennel seeds

1 teaspoon cumin seeds

1 teaspoon ground turmeric

1 teaspoon dried rose petals or buds

1 teaspoon dried rosemary

Place all the ingredients in an electric grinder or spice mill and grind to a fine powder. Store in an airtight jar away from light.

COOLING PUNGENT MASALA

PREP: 3 MINUTES   makes a little less than ¼ cup

It may sound like a contradiction, but this pungent spice blend has a cooling effect on the body. I learned it from Vaidya R. K. Mishra, whose father was very Fiery. He avoided heating foods but enjoyed this pungent masala even in the hottest days of summer without any aggravation. You can even sprinkle a couple of pinches on your tongue for a burst of *aaahhh*. Although well-tolerated by the Fiery, this spice blend is not for you if you have an acidic stomach.

4 teaspoons fennel seeds

4 teaspoons coriander seeds

1 teaspoon black peppercorns

1 teaspoon Sucanat, raw cane sugar, or coconut sugar

Place all the ingredients in an electric grinder or spice mill and grind to a fine powder. Store in an airtight jar away from light.

GROUNDING MASALA

PREP: 3 MINUTES   makes about ¼ cup

This spice blend is suitable for cold weather and Airy digestion. It increases the digestive fire and enhances circulation without overheating the body.

2 tablespoons coriander seeds

2 tablespoons fennel seeds

1 teaspoon ground turmeric

1 teaspoon cumin seeds

1 teaspoon whole cloves

1 teaspoon powdered sunthi ginger (see page 89; optional)

¾ teaspoon black peppercorns

Place all the ingredients in an electric grinder or spice mill and grind to a fine powder. Store in an airtight jar away from light.

DIGESTIVE MASALA

PREP: 3 MINUTES

This masala will not only invigorate a savory dish with its captivating aroma, but it will also make sure that no undigested residue is left behind in your gut. The kalonji seed, called "black seed" in the West, is one of the most researched spices today because it is highly effective and safe in addressing numerous chronic ailments such as hypertension, fungal infection, diabetes, and ulcers. Kalonji alone could be too hot for some people to handle; for this reason Vaidya R. K. Mishra created this synergistic blend to ensure the balance between the cleansing and calming effects of the spices on digestion. Add Digestive Masala at the beginning of cooking savory dishes like soups, vegetables, or leafy greens.

2 tablespoons coriander seeds

2 tablespoons fennel seeds

2 teaspoons cumin seeds

2 teaspoons kalonji seeds (aka black seed)

1 teaspoon ground turmeric

Place all the ingredients in an electric grinder or spice mill and grind to a fine powder. Store in an airtight jar away from light.

PART THREE

OUTFITTING YOUR NEW AYURVEDIC KITCHEN

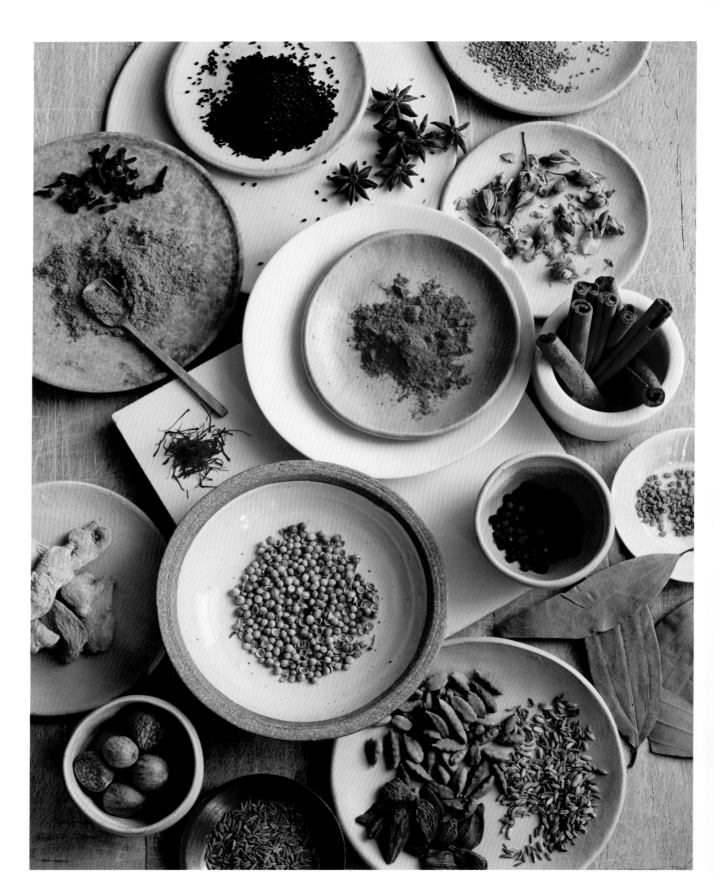

PLAYING WITH FLAVOR

WHY SPICES AND
HOW TO WORK WITH THEM

I meet a lot of people who tell me that when it comes to seasoning, salt and pepper is all they use. By the end of a cooking class, I introduce my students to at least ten other spices, and if our guests pass by my kitchen, they will see thirty more spice jars on the rack!

The art of seasoning foods is one of the most essential and subtle aspects of every cuisine. You could tell if a tomato was prepared Italian or Mexican style by the different condiments a cook used. Unfortunately, many cooks choose the fast way of flavoring by putting onions or garlic in (almost) everything and miss out on the captivating scenic route laid by upward of forty more spices.

With *What to Eat for How You Feel*, I want to take your seasoning skills to a whole new level. I want you to learn how to utilize herbs and spices not only for adding exquisite flavors, but for promoting health—balancing your elements, kindling your digestive fire, and eliminating impurities—and adding the six tastes to your meals.

Herbs and spices, like humans, are composed of the five elements. Dr. David Frawley explains in *The Yoga of Herbs* that each of the plant's tissues affects a corresponding tissue in the human body: the watery liquid of the plant works on liquid plasma; the sap works on blood; the soft part of the wood on muscle; the gum of the tree on fat; the bark on bone; the leaves on nerve tissue and bone marrow; and the flowers and fruits on the reproductive fluids. Seeds, which contain in unmanifest form all parts of the plant, work on the body as a whole.

The chemical makeup of spices can enhance or slow down our metabolic activities, helping or hindering them. That is why spices and herbs do not just contribute flavor to our palate; they are a necessary part of a healthy diet. They maintain our optimal metabolic rate, pacify our emotions, and clear mental fog through the balance of hormones and other chemicals that nourish our cells.

The ancients called spices and herbs "vehicles" equipped with the blueprints for healing. The minute they enter the body, they start to clean up the digestive tract, paving the way for nutrients to reach their final destination. Spices also help the body eliminate unwanted wastes in a timely manner. At times, these processes may slow down for us, and one reason could be that we are not eating food with sufficient spices.

Are You Spice Deficient?

Do you:

- feel tired after finishing a meal

- overeat because you don't feel satiated

- feel bloated

- experience acidity or heartburn

- feel sluggish

- get constipated

- crave sweets excessively after finishing a meal

If you do, your body is sending you signals of some imbalance in your digestive system. In the previous chapter, I shared spice blends that can help correct digestive imbalances.

How to Cook with Spices

As with food, when we use herbs and spices, we have to consider two things:

1. **Proper combination**—which spices properly combine with others and in what proportions

2. **Proper preparation**—how to cook them and in what medium

After years of studying curative cooking with spices, I still come across a "new" detail of what will work best for whom, how, and why. With proper combination and preparation, spices and herbs can help balance almost any kind of digestive ailment, correcting metabolic and assimilation problems. The art of cooking with spices is to use them just right—you don't want to be spice deficient, but you don't want to overdose on them either.

And don't forget to smell the spices! Even inhaling their aromas is therapeutic.

Spice Combinations

The essential principle of proper combination of spices is based not only on layering flavors but on balancing one spice's action with another. For example, the heating effect of turmeric, ginger, or chiles balances the cooling energy of fennel, coriander, cumin, cilantro, and dill, and vice versa. Get familiar with the spice combinations I use in the Grounding, Cooling, and Energizing recipes. Once you grasp the principle, you can easily create your own signature spice blends.

Cooking Methods

Every spice has volatile organic compounds (VOCs)—they make the spices' different aromas. The secret of cooking with spices is to use methods that protect their aroma and infuse their flavor into the food. The special nutrients of spices are mostly fat-soluble and water-soluble. It is important to use some oil and water with whatever you cook in order to provide the proper carriers for the spices' compounds. Exposing the spices to heat activates their inherent chemical properties, creating a molecular interaction between the spice and its medium (oil and water). Cooking makes the spices and herbs more easily available to our digestive system.

In *What to Eat for How You Feel*, I use the following cooking methods to awaken the aroma and medicinal properties of spices:

1. Ground or crushed into powder, added to a dish at the beginning of cooking.

2. Lightly toasted in a little oil at different stages of cooking.

3. Lightly toasted in a dry pan (toasting deactivates some of the pungency of the spice, making it less heating for the body; dry-toasting is often necessary to cool you down when you feel very Fiery).

4. Dry-toast individual spices to create a spice blend (known as masala)—these "precooked" spice blends are always best added at the end of cooking.

- You will further lock in the flavors if you cover your dish and let it simmer. Otherwise, at the end of cooking, your kitchen will smell great, but your food will be bland. That's a joke, but you get the idea.

- To substitute fresh herbs for dried herbs, a general rule is one to three: 1 teaspoon crumbled dried herbs equals 3 teaspoons (1 tablespoon) minced fresh herbs.

The Four Essential Spices for Cooking

Remember the time when you first set foot in the kitchen—what was the first dish you ever cooked? And what were the first spices you used? I honestly can't remember the first thing I ever cooked, but salt and pepper were definitely my firsts in the realm of seasoning. Many of us keep it simple and go with only salt and pepper for years.

If you are showing the symptoms of spice deficiency and decide to add more spice to your diet, these are the four essentials you may begin with: coriander, fennel, cumin, and turmeric. I call them "superspices" because of their wondrous healing properties (see "Properties of Spices" on page 232). If you are starting from scratch, get these four spices first and build up your spice rack gradually. And don't just let them sit on the shelf—use them daily!

Selection, Storage, and Shelf Life of Spices

SELECTING GOOD QUALITY

- Purchase non-irradiated and, if possible, organically grown herbs and spices (health food stores generally carry). You will find more options in the Sources section (page 250).

- Spices retain the greatest amount of flavorful essential oils when purchased whole and then are ground in a mortar and pestle or a small electric grinder just before using. Electric grinders work really well.

- Ground spices are not always 100 percent pure. Some manufacturers mix them with "fillers."

STORAGE

Herbs and spices are sensitive to fluctuations in temperature, moisture, and light. Ideal storage temperatures are 65°F to 73°F (18°C to 23°C), and relative humidity should not exceed 55°F (13°C). Light (indoor or sunlight) will strip your herbs and spices of their natural color and leach key nutrients. Therefore, purchase seasonings in small quantities and store them in airtight containers (glass is better than plastic) in a dry pantry, cupboard, or closet, not on the kitchen counter.

SHELF LIFE

If you store your herbs and whole spices properly, they will stay good and potent for up to a year. Freshly ground spice blends are best to use within a month or two if kept in airtight containers. Grind black peppercorns just before you cook with them, as they oxidize and turn acidic very quickly.

Preparing your own spice blends (masalas) is best—I have included a few recipes I love in the previous chapter. Make masalas in small quantities every four weeks to preserve their freshness and store as I suggest above.

About the Proper Use of Turmeric

It is the king, the chief, the champion among spices because its properties can support some of the most important functions of our physiology. Until the last decade or so, most people in Europe or the United States did not keep turmeric on their spice rack. Today, a growing number of positive scientific studies have made turmeric so desirable that it's available in every grocery store; every health food store now carries turmeric or curcumin capsules; every juice place offers fresh turmeric drinks. Nutritionists and health cooks add raw turmeric to their smoothies, cooking adventurists play with it until the food tastes good. It is exciting that science is validating turmeric's benefits, known to Ayurvedic practitioners for thousands of years. Modern research, however, still lacks the complete understanding of how to properly use turmeric. Some people think that if an herb is good for you, then you can mix it with anything, and the more the better. As with any spice that is so potent, turmeric's improper use can lead to negative results.

The ancients described turmeric as bitter, slightly pungent, heating, and drying. Its prime action on the body is detoxification by activating the liver, our main cleansing organ. Imagine turmeric as the best detergent for the central dishwasher of our organism. When our liver and blood are nice and clean, the rest of the body smiles.

Select the best quality if you want to get all the benefits. Real, freshly ground turmeric is of dark yellow-orange color with a strong pungent aroma. There is a lot of fake turmeric sold in the stores. The Food Fraud Database (www.foodfraud.org) lists dozens of shocking scientific reports on replacement ingredients in turmeric powder: starch, sawdust, synthetic dyes, clay, and more.

It is best to not take it raw in capsules, smoothies, salads, juices, or teas; do not sprinkle it on your salad. Fresh turmeric root contains all of its oils and properties in a crude form; as anything raw, it can be too harsh on the physiology. Vaidya R. K. Mishra writes in his article "The Magic of Turmeric Unveiled":

> When the liver starts to release toxins with the help of turmeric, and if the detox pathways found all over the body are not ready (they could be blocked, or incapable to handle a sudden toxic load efficiently), and if the other organs such as the kidneys, or the urinary tract, or the colon, have not been prepared to handle the release of large toxic loads, then the toxic waste being released by the liver all at once without previous preparation will surely result in a "detox crisis." If toxins do not find their way out of the body safely and effectively, they will get reabsorbed which can result in autoimmune conditions.

Traditionally in India, where people consume turmeric daily, turmeric was never eaten raw but only used after having being correctly dried in order to protect the liver from overheating.

Cook with it by adding some water and fat. The water, fat, and protein molecules will bind with the turmeric for a steady delivery to the cellular system, making sure that the liver does not get overwhelmed.

Add it at the beginning of cooking vegetables, lentils, or grains. You may also combine it with other spices and boil them with cow's milk, goat's milk, or almond milk. As I mentioned above, turmeric is drying and heating. To counteract the drying effect, we have to mix it with good fat, and to balance the heating effect, we have to combine it with cooling spices.

Combine it with cooling spices like coriander or fennel to pacify its heating potency. The Superspice Masala recipe (The Healing Properties of Spices, page 219) is a great way to be introduced to regular use of turmeric.

Use in moderation, starting with pinches when introducing it in your diet. Cut back if you show signs of detox crisis, such as diarrhea or skin rash. For a regular dose, ¼ to ½ teaspoon turmeric powder per person per meal is enough.

It is important for very Fiery individuals to limit turmeric, especially in the summer. When you are too heated or the weather is hot, you may consume turmeric by cooking it in coconut oil (¼ teaspoon turmeric in 1 tablespoon coconut oil). Sauté it over very low heat for 15 seconds, then drizzle it on food. Common symptoms of turmeric overdose are constipation, diarrhea, and skin rash.

Contraindications: Turmeric is not recommended when there is high fever, active hemorrhoids, or tuberculosis. If you are on any medication (including blood thinners) or are experiencing serious health problems, check with your medical doctor before using turmeric.

An Overview of the Metabolic Effects and Healing Properties of Spices and Herbs

These are the herbs and spices I use in the recipes of this book. I am listing but a few of their many healing properties.

SPICE / HERB	PREDOMINANT TASTE / METABOLIC EFFECT	HEALING PROPERTIES
Ajwain	Pungent/very heating	Increases appetite, stimulates digestion, eliminates toxins, relieves congestion, clears the taste buds; "fertilizer" for friendly bacteria to grow
Asafoetida	Pungent /very heating	Increases appetite, aids digestion, decreases abdominal pain and bloating
Basil	Sweet, pungent, astringent/slightly heating	Relieves coughs, colds, headaches, fevers; improves immunity, opens circulatory channels
Bay leaf	Sweet, pungent, astringent/slightly heating	Improves digestion, decreases abdominal pain and bloating, diuretic
Black pepper	Pungent/heating	Improves digestion, opens circulatory channels, eliminates toxins, liquefies hard mucus, enhances oxygenation in the channels of the brain
Black seed (kalonji)	Pungent/heating	Supports digestion, enhances flavor and absorption, reduces mucus and bloating, antibacterial, purifies uterus, regulates hormonal system
Cardamom (black)	Pungent/heating	Improves sluggish digestion, enhances protein metabolism, eliminates toxins
Cardamom (green)	Sweet, pungent/cooling	Calms nerves, aids digestion, freshens mouth, helps with protein metabolism and chronic cough
Cassia leaf (tej patta)	Sweet, pungent/slightly heating	Improves circulation, relieves coughs and colds, helps with glucose and carbohydrate metabolism
Chile, green Thai	Pungent/very heating	Improves circulation, decreases congestion, burns toxins
Cilantro	Sweet, astringent/cooling	Reduces acidity, improves digestion, heavy-metal detoxifier, diuretic
Cinnamon	Sweet, pungent/heating	Improves circulation, relieves coughs and colds, helps with glucose and carbohydrate metabolism
Clove	Pungent/slightly heating	Improves digestion, reduces toxins and congestion, soothes coughs, opens circulatory channels
Coriander	Sweet, astringent/cooling	Improves digestion, offsets spicy foods, relieves gas, diuretic, calms the mind, binds toxins in the blood, protects from acidity
Cumin	Pungent, astringent/slightly heating	Stimulates digestion, eliminates toxins, relieves congestion, helps with absorption of nutrients, "fertilizer" for friendly bacteria to grow

SPICE / HERB	PREDOMINANT TASTE / METABOLIC EFFECT	HEALING PROPERTIES
Curry leaf	Sweet, astringent/cooling	Supports liver detox, purifies the blood, manages cholesterol and blood sugar, cleanses the cellular system
Dill	Bitter, astringent/cooling	Relieves spasms, stops growth of various bacteria, yeast, and mold; soothes colic in babies
Fennel	Sweet, astringent/cooling (in smaller amounts; heating in large amounts)	Regulates digestive fire—increases weak fire and decreases overly strong fire, promotes breast milk flow, estrogenic
Fenugreek	Pungent, bitter/heating	Promotes breast milk flow, strengthens bones, regulates sugar and fat metabolism, supports the stamina of the liver and pancreas
Ginger	Pungent/very heating	Improves digestion and circulation, breaks down fat in the stomach, relieves constipation; reduces mucus, and inflammation; antiviral and antibacterial; also see page 89
Mace	Pungent, astringent, Sour/heating	Kindles digestive fire
Mint	Sweet/cooling	Soothes the stomach, improves digestion
Mustard seed	Pungent/very heating	Improves sluggish digestion, clears sinuses
Nutmeg	Sweet, astringent, pungent/slightly heating	Calms the mind, promotes sleep, relieves coughs and colds, decreases morning sickness, stops diarrhea, supports men's energy, increases absorption in the colon
Oregano	Pungent/very heating	Antibacterial, antifungal, antiviral, calms the nervous system
Parsley	Astringent, pungent/slightly heating	Blood purifier, stimulates the bowels, diuretic, reduces inflammation in kidneys, antifungal, builds blood, stimulates brain activity
Rose buds/petals	Sweet/cooling	Soothes the heart, balances the mind, slows down aging; rejuvenates the digestive tract, liver, and colon; promotes glowing skin
Rosemary	Astringent, sweet/slightly heating	Beneficial for headaches, eases menstruation, antioxidant, anti-inflammatory, boosts immune system, improves blood circulation, helps digestion, prevents brain aging
Saffron	Sweet, astringent, bitter/heating	Purifies blood, improves digestion, calms nerves, helps prevent Parkinson's disease, supports the heart
Thyme	Pungent/heating	Soothes coughs, improves digestion, decreases gas
Turmeric	Bitter, pungent, astringent/heating	Cleanses the liver, breaks down fat in the liver, improves digestion and immunity, anti-inflammatory; antioxidant, adds luster to the skin, stops bleeding; also see pages 230-231
Vanilla	Sweet, astringent/cooling	Aphrodisiac, improves appetite

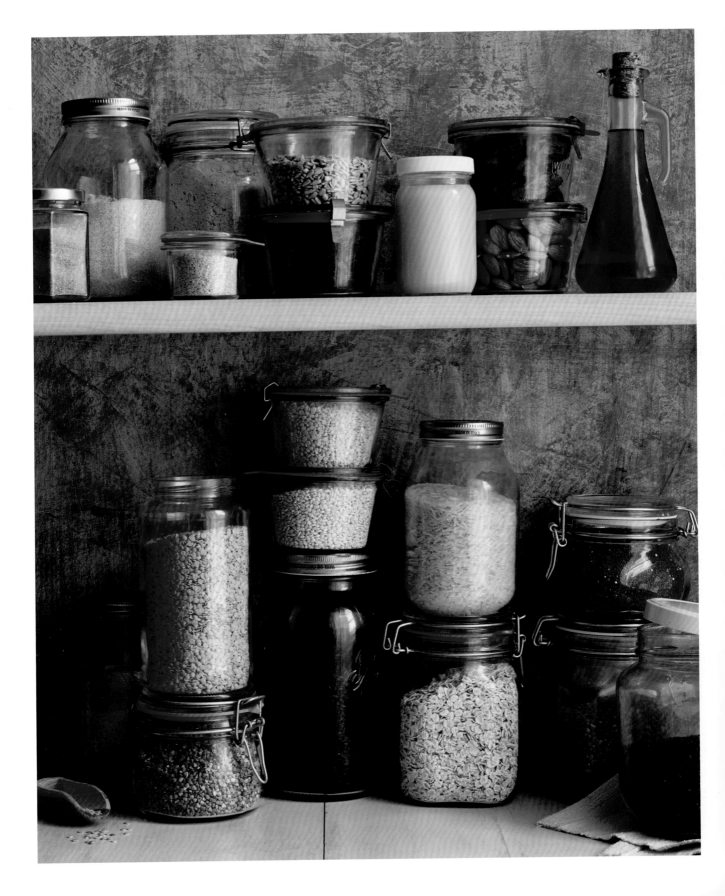

CHOOSING FOODS
FOR YOUR NEW
AYURVEDIC KITCHEN

Over the past few decades, our food has become canned, bleached, refined, chemically preserved, pasteurized, sterilized, homogenized, hydrogenated, artificially colored, de-fibered, highly sugared, highly salted, synthetically fortified (enriched), genetically modified, and generally exposed to hundreds of new manmade chemicals. When our food is corrupted like that, our cells start acting less intelligently. Why let such denatured foods clutter your pantry, and then your body and your mind?

There is no doubt that for food to grant us its highest benefits, it has to be of the highest quality, i.e., the way God or nature designed it in the first place. Fresh, locally grown, seasonal, organic, wholesome (unprocessed), invigorating—such quality ingredients will support your body in doing all the intelligent things it is designed to do.

Here is the list of ingredients generally favored in SV Ayurvedic cooking, most of which I have used in the recipes of this book. I also outline a list of foods popular in health-conscious circles that I prefer to avoid and why. I am aware that often the best quality comes at the highest cost. If you are on a small budget, look for the next best not only in price but also in quality. Eating better quality, more vibrant food pays off with better health (and lower medical bills) in the long run.

Stocking Your New Ayurvedic Pantry

Oils/Fats: Organic cultured ghee and butter (ideally grass-fed), extra-virgin coconut oil, extra-virgin olive oil, sesame oil, black sesame oil

Dairy: Organic, grass-fed, raw or unhomogenized, full-fat milk; yogurt, buttermilk

Grains: Basmati rice (white), quinoa, amaranth, barley, millet, buckwheat, oats; occasionally red rice, black rice (aka forbidden rice), wild rice, fresh non-GMO corn; pasta (quinoa, lentil, einkorn)

Flours: Organic, whole flours from einkorn, spelt, farro (emmer), kamut, quinoa, amaranth, buckwheat, barley, rye, oats, besan (small chickpeas), teff, sorghum (freshly ground flour is the healthiest, as it provides the highest nutrition, flavor, taste, and digestibility)

Legumes: Small beans: mung, adzuki, black chickpeas (aka kala chana), kulthi (aka horse gram; see page 69)

Lentils: yellow split mung dal, red, black, green, French; chana dal (small split chickpeas)

Fruits: All sweet and juicy fruits; dried fruits

Vegetables: All except nightshades (potatoes, tomatoes, eggplants, peppers), onions, garlic

Seeds and nuts: All except for peanuts; raw, unsalted; coconut

Sweeteners: Date sugar, coconut (palm) sugar, raw cane sugar, Sucanat, raw honey, maple syrup, fructose

Spices: Almost all spices; organic, non-irradiated

Fresh herbs and condiments: All fresh herbs; green Thai chiles, ginger, curry leaves (see page 172) , lemongrass, Kaffir lime leaves; Soma Salt (see page 46), Himalayan rock salt, Real Salt

Ingredients I Avoid in My Recipes

Unlike modern nutrition, Ayurveda considers not only the effects of what you eat today; it also looks at how the food you eat today could affect your whole life. Some foods may provide immediate benefits to the body, but their regular daily use may lead to imbalance in the long term. This is a list of ingredients I chose not to use in my recipes and why.

Meat, fish, and eggs: Although Ayurveda describes all categories of foods, including meat, fish, and eggs, the consumption of these foods is prescribed for specific conditions rather than recommended for daily indulgence. According to the words of the sages, the lacto-vegetarian diet is considered most conducive for people on a spiritual path, as this diet involves the least cruelty to other living beings and opens the heart to experience the deepest levels of compassion. Eggs, although used by a lot of vegetarian cooks and in most vegetarian cookbooks, are embryos, and avoiding eggs, especially fertilized ones, is yet another act of nonviolence. Eggs also are an acid-forming food. Whether for ethical, economic, environmental, religious, or health reasons, eating or not eating animal protein is a personal choice. For more than two decades I have abstained from meat, fish, and eggs for all the above reasons; therefore I do not use them in my recipes. I incorporate high-quality dairy as the least cruel source of animal protein.

Onions, garlic, and their allium cousins:
Avoid these? This is shocking news, especially because most of the Ayurvedic cookbooks use them. Garlic is a powerful herb, and SV Ayurvedic doctors use it as medicine but do not recommend it as food for daily consumption. Because it is a broad-spectrum antibiotic, garlic (especially raw) kills not only the bad germs but also the most needed friendly bacteria. Garlic does not discriminate between the "bad guys" and the "good guys" in your gut. Raw onions are a stimulating and very heating food. Cooked onions and garlic have less of an effect (both therapeutic and harmful), because cooking destroys much of the sulfur they contain. Yet enough of it remains to still harm the friendly bacteria in your gut, especially if you are among the majority of people who lack a good environment for the bacteria to thrive. If you are one of the few blessed with lots of friendly bacteria and keep a good routine and diet, then whether onions and garlic are good for you depends on how much and how frequently you consume them and what other foods you eat to buffer and balance their negative properties. For example, if you consume onions or garlic (both very heating) with cooling vegetables such as summer squash, and if you are not a Fiery type, your colon might handle the excess sulfur content without trouble and your friendly bacteria will not be harmed.

On an energetic level, onions and garlic constrict the energy channels, thus preventing a person from experiencing mental clarity and higher states of consciousness. Vaidya Mishra once told me that whoever eats garlic and onion will have very strong body, but their spiritual antennas will be blocked. I stopped eating alliums more than twenty-six years ago because of my yoga practice. Referring to the ancient texts about yoga, my teachers advised me that if I wanted to succeed in meditation, I had to avoid foods that are overly stimulating or clouding to the mind.

If you feel overheated; if you like to do yoga, chant, or meditate; if you want mental clarity or balanced emotions, then a diet without onions and garlic may greatly support your spiritual practice. If you have eaten them your whole life, why not experiment without them for a month and see how you feel?

Nightshades—potato, tomato, eggplant, and peppers: I know I am stepping on a lot of people's toes when I say that it is better to reduce or avoid eating nightshades. I grew up in Bulgaria, a small country famous for its export of incredible tomatoes and peppers. People there—and in Italy and Mexico—eat tomatoes at practically every meal. And try to convince a German or an Irish person to stop eating potatoes! Potatoes are among the largest crops in every country; people are eating them all over the world and doing just fine, so why avoid them?

One of the main reasons is that nightshades contain the following neurotoxins: nicotine, atropine, chaconine, tomatine, solanine, and scopolamine. These toxins may cause or sustain nerve damage or inflammation of joints and muscles. They also block the subtle energy channels. That is why nightshades are excluded from anti-inflammatory and pain-reducing diets and from healing cuisines such as macrobiotic and SV Ayurvedic diets.

Soy products: The most recent research on soy gives us good reasons to avoid it, even in fermented foods such as miso and tempeh. Most of the soy in the United States that's not organic is genetically modified, which makes it extremely allergenic and inflammatory. It is also known that soy inhibits thyroid function and can lead to hormonal problems because it mimics estrogen in humans. Soy enhances copper absorption in the liver and may lead to liver cell damage. It also blocks zinc uptake, and deficiency of zinc can also increase copper levels and toxicity. In general, soy is very hard to digest, and difficult-to-digest food is another way to make the body toxic.

Yeasts (such as nutritional yeast, active dry yeast, brewer's yeast): These are fungi that generate toxins in the gut. They also encourage the growth of *Candida albicans*, which wrecks havoc in the body. Yeasted breads are quite constipating.

Canned foods (including coconut milk and almond milk): They are often treated with chemicals to preserve a fresh look and extend shelf life. Although there may be some nutrients left, the prana of canned food is completely gone, making it "dead" and very difficult to digest. Instead of giving you energy, canned food will take energy away from you. The toxic substances in the can material themselves present yet other problem.

Refined, processed, and artificial foods: These include refined sugar, flours, and pasta. During the refining process, sugar and flours are bleached and they lose their total nutritional value and prana. As they are low on fiber, they also are very constipating. Processed foods are also more likely to trigger allergic reactions.

Polyunsaturated fats: These include canola, safflower, sunflower, corn, peanut, soybean, and other vegetable oils. They are often genetically modified and contaminated with toxic solvents used in production. These oils are unstable for cooking, easily oxidize, and therefore may cause or sustain inflammation.

Modern wheat (red, hard, white): Modern wheat has been so heavily hybridized and modified that its molecular weight of proteins and starch is much higher than what many people can digest. One reason many people today (especially in the United States) react to wheat is because if it is not organic, modern wheat is hybridized so as to be able to withstand applications of Roundup, a powerful patented herbicide that is designed to kill all plants, including weeds, that haven't been bred to survive it. Fields of crops are sprayed with Roundup, which kills the weeds—but remains on the surviving wheat. The main ingredient in this weed killer is glyphosate, which has been scientifically linked to cause digestive disorders, leaky gut, infertility, and many more health problems. And of course the Roundup Ready wheat has a modified genome, not its ancient one. Because genetic cross-contamination from organic to nonorganic crops in wheat fields happens quite often, I decided to totally replace modern wheat with its original ancestor, einkorn, which has never been hybridized and is much easier to digest. Spelt, farro, and kamut are other options, although they are hybrids and heavier for the gut.

Brown rice: Most Ayurvedic practitioners recommend white basmati rice as the most medicinal of all rice varieties. It is sweet in taste, cooling, strengthening, easily digestible, aphrodisiac, strengthens the body, and helps to clear taste and voice. When eaten in moderation, it balances every body type.

Brown rice is more nutritious, yes, but is it healthier for you? It all depends on your digestion: if your digestive fire is strong enough to break down the fiber-rich husk of brown rice, then you may enjoy more of it, especially in the winter. However, if you have sluggish digestion and slow metabolism, then eating brown rice may produce semidigested toxins that can cause havoc in your gut. If you feel tired after eating brown rice, your digestion is probably not strong enough to handle it.

Fermented cheeses: see page 204.

Coffee: There are many contradicting opinions on whether coffee is good for you. In terms of qualities, coffee is bitter, drying, acidic, stimulating, but ultimately depleting to the system. I like Dr. John Douillard's analogy in *The 3-Season Diet*: "It's a little like borrowing money from the bank to get through the month, but never earning any money to pay back the loan." Borrowing non-food energy from large amounts of coffee could ultimately lead to adrenal insufficiency, an imbalance in which our adrenal hormones are exhausted from constant stress. If you don't want to give up coffee, try these tips to minimize its unwanted effects: 1) use the best quality organic beans (nonorganic are loaded with pesticides); 2) find quality beans that are free from mold (some coffee bean harvests develop mold at their place of origin, even before being shipped to sellers); 3) never drink coffee on empty stomach; 4) brew it with a cardamom pod to reduce acidity. Or look for coffee substitutes such as Vaidya's Cup (available at www.chandika.com), which is a superior coffee alternative—invigorating, alkalizing, tasty, and even cleansing for the liver and kidneys.

Chocolate: Although full of polyphenols and antioxidants that fight free radicals, the nature of cocoa beans is acidic, heating, drying, and clogging. Typical chocolate bars have added sugar, soy, dairy, and artificial flavors. Like coffee, cocoa is also very prone to mold contamination. If I were to enjoy chocolate once in a while, I'd buy a chocolate that's at least 85 percent dark or, even better, prepare a recipe chocolate-based myself, adding spices like pink pepper and cinnamon to counteract cocoa's clogging properties. It is best to enjoy chocolate only occasionally.

Flax seeds and oil: They may be a showcase of omega-3 fatty acids, but they are among the most heating substances on the planet, and Ayurveda recommends them only for severe Airy imbalance. Regular use of flax seeds could lead to different symptoms of Fiery imbalance, including overheated liver and spleen. Since most of us are victims of a stressful lifestyle and polluted environment that overheat the liver and other organs, I choose to avoid flax.

Cayenne (dried) and fresh red chiles: With their sharp and harsh fiery nature, they could dry the moist lining of the stomach and generate hyperacidity. Green Thai chiles have a little less heat and more moisture, making them a more balancing source of pungent taste.

Table salt: It has been refined and stripped down of all minerals but sodium, then "enriched" with fillers and aluminum anticaking agents. Iodized salt does not nearly provide you with the recommended daily doze of iodine. According to Ayurveda, the best salt is Soma Salt (aka *saindhava*) or white Himalayan rock salt. Otherwise, pink Himalayan salt, Real Salt, and sea salt are better options than processed table salt.

Vinegar: Lowers the body's pH, making it acidic and less immune. It also contains large amounts of yeast and fungal residue. Apple cider vinegar is an exception, but because Ayurveda considers it of low pranic value, I prefer to avoid it in my cooking. Lime is a great substitute and source of sour taste.

Alcohol: Besides being a highly addictive intoxicating substance, alcohol is extremely heating and acid-forming, and it will give you food cravings, brain fog, and reduced immunity. It is a liquid of highly concentrated sugar, so it also negatively affects one's blood sugar levels. Ayurveda sometimes prescribes herbal wine remedies to be taken in very small doses, not for recreational drinking. Wine (especially organic and aged) may help you digest heavy foods like meat, but it is often contaminated with mold toxins and triggers yeast growth. Hard liquor is the most damaging alcohol to the body.

Fermented vegetables: Ayurveda uses fermentation for the preparation of numerous foods and remedies. The Vedic tradition is to pickle foods of sour taste such as lime, lemon, orange, and mango and use them as digestive aids. Keep in mind that any fermented foods are too heating for when you're experiencing acidic Fiery digestion.

Lemon: It's a good citrus, but I prefer to use lime when a sour taste is needed because lemon is more sharp and acidic and it takes longer to turn alkaline in the body; many of us today need less acidic foods to stay balanced.

Winter squash: Pumpkin, butternut squash, acorn squash, spaghetti squash, kabocha squash, and other orange-flesh squashes are delicious and nutritious, but they are hard to digest, and their dry and heavy nature may eventually create blockages in the circulatory channels throughout the body. Sweet potato is a good substitute.

Mushrooms: They are technically fungi, and according to Ayurveda, as a food they are hard to digest and aggravate every body type. If you choose to eat mushrooms, the white ones have less damaging effects.

Leftovers: I am very sorry to say that after four hours of preparation, food, even when refrigerated, begins to decompose and lose its prana. The longer the time gap between cooking food and eating it, the less its medicinal value; leftover food is much harder to digest. Have you noticed how sluggish you feel after finishing off the holiday leftovers? Cooking meals on Sunday, freezing them, and eating them throughout the week could save you time, but it will gradually diminish your health. Try chopping vegetables on Sunday for quick cooking during the week instead. According to SV Ayurveda, the most toxic leftovers are beans and lentils because four hours after they've been cooked their starch turns into an indigestible starch that leads to gas and bloating, especially when you're feeling Airy. The popular belief that bean dishes are better when cooked the day before and refrigerated does not hold true on the level of healthy digestion.

The best way to move away from the foods on the "avoid" list is to introduce new, delicious recipes into your diet and experiment with foods you may have never tried before. Cooking with flavor-enhancing spices also helps. With a little attention and practice, you will be satisfied with food without stressing over it and running the risk of causing blockages in your system.

THE
DAIRY QUESTION

The alarming increase of conditions associated with dairy consumption—allergies, inflammation, autoimmune disorders, osteoporosis, arthritis, heart disease, cancer—has stirred numerous discussions and produced research resulting in controversial and contradictory opinions. It is really confusing, especially when a strong theory is aggressively challenged a few years later. To me, the Ayurvedic perspective makes the most sense; I will briefly present it in this chapter because I do use dairy products in some of my recipes as a good vegetarian source of protein. Why? For a number of reasons.

Protein is built from amino acids found in two dietary categories: vegetable and animal. In terms of molecular structure, the three-dimensional shape of animal protein differs from that of vegetable protein; that means that biochemically the two types of protein behave differently in the human body. Deficiency in even one of the essential amino acids results in degradation of the body's proteins (bone, muscle, enzymes, cells). Such deficiency often leads to high heat or acidity imbalance, especially in the bones and muscles. Sensitive teeth and receding tooth enamel are symptoms of such imbalance.

Complete proteins are best supplied through food daily, and therefore we need to include both vegetable and animal protein in our daily meals. Legumes, whole grains, nuts, seeds, and some vegetables are an excellent source of vegetable protein. The only source of animal protein for lacto-vegetarians remains dairy products like milk, yogurt, and fresh cheese. Therefore, especially if you are a vegetarian, yes, you do need dairy in your diet. I followed a vegan diet for a while, and can sympathize with the choice to abstain from any kind of animal products, be it because of allergies or for ethical reasons. Staying balanced on a vegan diet, without any dairy, can be challenging, but it is achievable with effort.

Are Humans Supposed to Drink the Milk of Another Animal?

One of the eternal laws of nature is that one living being is food for another. We human beings are naturally omnivores, eating both plants and animals, and even more versatile in what we can eat because of our ability to cook and make food easier to digest.

More than five thousand years ago, the Indian sages who wrote the Vedas stated that grains, fruits, vegetables, and milk are the recommended ingredients for an enlightened human diet. Today many people in India still consider the cow holy and take care of her as part of the family. In Vedic culture the cow is regarded as our mother because she generously gives six to seven gallons of milk daily. That's a lot of milk, way more than her calf can drink! Once the calf has drunk to its heart's content, humans have to empty the cow's udder (or else she would die) and put the milk to use. That was the understanding and practice in cultures throughout the world, not only India, for centuries.

Now, whether consuming dairy is good for you personally is another question. For many people today, it isn't. In this case, we have to follow the law of common sense.

History has proven that milk can be safe to consume for millions of people; people have thrived with dairy products for thousands of years. We can't ignore this fact. But why are so many people today having problems with it? And why are dairy allergies so common today but were hardly spoken of fifty years ago?

From an Ayurvedic perspective, there are three main reasons: 1) conventional dairy production, 2) our weakened digestive systems, and 3) improper dairy consumption.

Research supports the opinions of many holistic health practitioners that conventional milk produced in the last few decades has caused a rise of dairy intolerance. Even without the research, to me it is common sense. The living conditions at factory farm dairies are far different from the cow's natural habitat. Instead of happily grazing in the fields, the cows are forced to live in confinement and ingest pesticide-loaded grains, antibiotics, and synthetic growth hormones; the cows are treated harshly and never have the space to properly bond with their calves—all these ways of mistreating a cow affect the quality of her milk. Such milk is certainly harmful, as is clearly evident from the numerous medical studies on conventional milk consumption. Please note that most, if not all, research on dairy consumption has been conducted on conventional milk only.

Many people turn to a vegan diet not only for health reasons but because they do not want to support the cruel and non-ecological practices of conventional farming. Unfortunately, wherever there is commercialization and a profit-based economy, unethical exploitation is inevitable. Not only the production of cow's milk but almost every aspect of life is tainted with some form of violence.

Simple abstaining from cow's milk by a few is more of a reactive approach that will not likely have much impact in helping the suffering cows. A more effective and lasting solution would be to promote cow protection through positive education. Fortunately, compassionate farms do exist all over the world—even though small in number, they set a wonderful example of sustainable agriculture and of treating our friends the animals and Mother Earth with love and care.

Lactose intolerance also causes problems with dairy consumption. One is unable to digest lactose when one's gut does not release sufficient quantity of the enzyme lactase. If you are lactose intolerant by birth, there is not much you can do about it. Most people, however, develop this intolerance over time: the digestive system weakens because of so many reasons—consuming low-quality milk in the wrong way, stress, an unnatural lifestyle, to name a few; sometimes genetic predisposition plays a role. The large intestine gradually loses its ability to release enough lactase to fully digest the lactose; the semidigested lactose begins to putrefy in the colon and turns into toxins that then are reabsorbed in the body, harming the immune system. I was able to clear this type of lactose intolerance with consistent SV Ayurvedic and Nambudripad's Allergy Elimination Techniques (NAET) treatments.

Milk Glossary

There are a few important terms to understand when talking about milk:

Ahimsa: *Ahimsa* is a Sanskrit word with many connotations, but its root meaning is basically "nonviolence" or "without harm." It is used to refer to milk from cows that are happy and loved and will never be killed. Such milk is rather rare to find because even the organic dairy farms send their cows to slaughter when they grow too old to produce milk. Nevertheless, throughout the world there are compassionate no-kill farms with Adopt-a-Cow programs.

Organic: Refers to milk from cows not treated with synthetic hormones and antibiotics or fed with GMO and pesticide-loaded grains.

Grass-fed/pasture-raised: Refers to milk from cows fed their natural food—grass and hay.

A study conducted by the USDA has determined that pasture-fed cows produce milk containing as much as five times the level of conjugated linoleic acid (CLA), a known anti-carcinogen, as cows managed in confined housing.

Conventional: Refers to milk produced in factory farms where the cows are often mistreated, fed unnatural GMO grains (and even chicken beaks, junk food, or sawdust!), injected with hormones and antibiotics, and brutally slaughtered as soon as they stop giving milk.

Raw: Refers to unprocessed milk with all its nutrients, bacteria, and proteins preserved. Currently, ten states allow the retail sale of raw milk. In the rest of the United States, sales regulations vary. Check www.farmto-consumer.org for details. Uncooked raw milk is best digested when it is still warm and frothy, immediately after milking the cow. Refrigerated raw milk is best digested when boiled, ideally with spices. Make sure the farm you're getting your raw milk from follows proper farming and hygiene standards.

Pasteurized: Pasteurization is a process of heating milk at high temperature to reduce the risk of milk contamination with pathogens and to extend its shelf life. The process denatures milk proteins and makes casein (milk's primary protein) difficult to digest. It also destroys lactase, the enzyme that helps us digest lactose, reduces the vitamin content in the milk, and makes its calcium difficult for a human body to absorb. Avoid the ultrapasteurized milk.

Homogenized: Homogenization is the processing of milk by breaking down (and damaging) its fats and distributing them throughout the milk so that the cream is permanently mixed in, which extends its shelf life. The larger and differentiated fat globules in raw milk hold the nutrients and lactose and cause slower absorption in the gut because they're more complex to break down. The faster absorption of homogenized milk is more shocking to the digestive system and can lead to greater chance of lactose intolerance and inflammation.

Non-homogenized: Also labeled as "cream on top" or "creamline"; refers to milk that is pasteurized but not homogenized; available in health food stores across the country.

Fortified: Refers to pasteurized milk with added vitamins A and D. These vitamins are often synthetic, and according to some natural health practitioners, the body treats them as toxins.

Whole: Refers to full-fat milk, closest to the way it comes from the cow.

Low-fat or skim (nonfat): Refers to milk that is processed to reduce or eliminate fat. Such milk is much harder to digest. A lot of the milk's nutrients are lipid-soluble, so removing the fat from the milk also lowers its essential nutrient content. Regular consumption of low-fat milk is associated with osteopenia (thin bones) and osteoporosis (very frail bones).

Colostrum: The milk a cow gives immediately after giving birth. Ayurveda recommends that during the first week after birth, the colostrum milk should be reserved for the baby calf only—it is its rightful claim.

The Three Rules for Proper Milk Consumption

Milk is the basic dairy product that gets transformed into other forms of dairy such as yogurt, cheese, butter, buttermilk, or ghee. Here I will focus on milk; you will learn about the other dairy products in The New Ayurvedic Kitchen Staples chapter (pages 200 to 223).

Ayurveda calls milk "ambrosia," but when consumed in the wrong way, it can turn into poison for the body. Drinking milk in the wrong way will sooner or later lead to allergies or inflammation. To make milk the least harmful and get its ambrosial benefits, there are three factors to consider: quality, compatibility, and consumption.

1. Quality: Not All Milk Is the Same

Choose the best quality dairy whenever possible: Ahimsa, raw, whole, organic, from grass-fed cows. Since this quality is rather difficult to find, search for the next best: organic, whole, unhomogenized; try to stick to organic and whole milk at all costs. Many of us get negative reactions from eating conventional dairy. Honestly, if I had to choose between consuming conventional dairy and avoiding dairy completely, I'd choose the latter. Conventional dairy is just too unnatural for our bodies.

2. Compatibility: Mixing Milk with Other Foods

As I discussed in "Opposites That Don't Attract" (pages 36 to 40), milk only combines well with foods of sweet taste, such as grains, nuts, and dates. To protect your digestion, avoid mixing milk or cream with sour foods, salt, meat, fish, radishes, bananas, other raw fruits, nightshades, sesame seeds, cheese, or yogurt in either an individual dish or a meal.

3. Consumption: How and When You Eat It

By nature, milk is heavy to digest and therefore more likely to cause congestion and phlegm. Drinking cold-out-of-the-fridge milk makes it extra clogging. If you wish to drink cool milk, boil it first and then cool it to room temperature. You can further limit milk's phlegm-increasing tendencies by boiling it for five minutes with appropriate spices (see the recipes on pages 135 and 183).

BASIC KITCHEN EQUIPMENT FOR YOUR NEW AYURVEDIC KITCHEN

The kitchen is the place where you and food go on a date. Your kitchen doesn't have to be big and fancy; it's the atmosphere that counts. When you bring your unique individual presence into your cooking space, that energy will charge whatever food you prepare there.

Of course, you need some basic equipment to cook. Equipping your kitchen is a gradual and long-term investment. Once you buy a pan or a pot, it can last for decades. If you are starting a kitchen from scratch, get the good-quality essentials first, and then piece by piece add more appliances or gadgets. The main principle is to make your kitchen comfortable and practical, a space you love to be in.

Here are a few points to consider when you select your kitchen equipment. In general, I like to keep things simple and make sure that I can fit everything in my kitchen.

What is it made from: Avoid pots and utensils made from reactive, toxic materials such as aluminum, nonstick surfaces, glazed clay pots (they often contain lead), and plastic. Unglazed clay pots are traditional in Ayurvedic cooking and are my favorite among the most natural cooking vessels, but they may not be most practical or easy for you to get used to. Clay is a porous material. The pores of a clay pot allow the heated water in it to pass through as steam. In this way, the food retains its moisture, flavor, and nutrients. Other good materials are glass, ceramic, stone, well-seasoned cast iron, and high-quality stainless steel. See Sources (page 250) for suggested brands and stores.

Size: Select the size of your pots and pans according to the number of people you usually cook for—if you mostly cook just for yourself, then you need 1½- to 3-quart pans and pots. Standard cookware sets are suitable for a small family of two to four.

Quality: Save yourself the unnecessary frustration from buying poor-quality cookware. In the long run, it costs more. Cheap utensils break or corrode faster, and their makeup often includes unhealthy materials such as aluminum. If you cannot afford the highest quality equipment, go for medium grade.

Essential Tools

Adjust pot, pan, and bowl sizes according to your usual volume of cooking.

CUTTING/SLICING/CRUSHING

- **A chef's knife, a paring knife, a serrated knife**
- **A wooden cutting board**
- **A grater**
- **A peeler**
- **A mortar and pestle** (to grind herbs and spices)

MEASURING

- **A set of stainless steel measuring spoons**
- **A set of stainless steel measuring cups**
- **A glass 4-cup measuring cup**

COOKING

- **A 1½-quart and two 3- to 4-quart saucepans with lids**
- **A 10- to 12-inch heavy sauté pan with a lid**
- **A well-seasoned 10-inch cast-iron skillet** (the natural nonstick)
- **One or two baking sheets: 9 x 13 inches, 13 x 18 inches**
- **Baking pans: muffin pans, 8 x 8-inch glass pans, a 1½-pound loaf pan**
- **A steamer or a steaming basket**
- **Three mixing bowls: small, medium, large** (stainless steel or glass)
- **Two or three mixing and serving spoons** (wooden and stainless steel)
- **A soup ladle**
- **Spatulas** (rubber, wooden, and stainless steel)
- **Two-pronged fork for fluffing grains**

STRAINING

- **A set of mesh strainers** (small, medium, large)
- **A colander**
- **Cheesecloth** (to press cheese)
- **Nut milk bag** (to squeeze fresh nut milks)

Essential Electric Appliances

These appliances will speed up your cooking and increase the variety of recipes you can prepare.

- **A spice or coffee grinder** (to grind spices and nuts)
- **A blender** (to finely puree soups and drinks; to make nut milks)
- **A food processor** (to save time and energy chopping, grinding, and grating)
- **A pressure cooker** (to save cooking time—up to 70 percent, especially when cooking legumes)
- **A slow cooker** (to prepare one-pot meals overnight or while away from the kitchen)
- **A grain mill**

CONCLUSION:
Cooking as a Path to Awakening

With *What to Eat for How You Feel*, I have taken you on a journey of discovering a new relationship with food. It is a path of awakening and unfolding, where you learn to understand which foods are right for you; where you try new recipes and enjoy delicious meals; and where you are encouraged to notice the effects of food on your body and mind, which can motivate you to choose more of the foods that make you feel better. There is an energetic thread that connects the food you put in your body both to its original source and to its ultimate transformation into physical and mental energy. Expanding your awareness of how everything is connected is one of the aspects of yoga, which literally means "to link." The sister sciences yoga and Ayurveda have long been connected; they are two parts of a world view that has guided humans to health and wholeness for thousands of years and can guide us on our path with food and in the kitchen as well.

Yoga directly relates to Ayurveda because the two were designed to work together. They are like the two tracks on the railroad of the human journey. Practicing one without the other is incomplete and rather difficult. Practicing them together speeds up advancement and brings fulfillment. However, if yoga is not your calling, any kind of practice that increases awareness of the personal connectedness of all beings and things will nurture your positive attitude, respect, and higher intentions.

In whatever ways you express your spirituality, please consider concluding your cooking as I have learned to do, with a blessing of the food and a prayer of thanks. For me, a blessing helps me connect with the source of food and express my gratitude to the Creator, nature, and to everyone who contributed to my meal. Acting with such sense of connectedness is the essence of yoga. By bringing yoga into your kitchen, culinary art transforms into a path to spiritual awakening—your way to commune with divinity and humanity through food.

My cooking journey began in the kitchen of a yoga ashram. Cleanliness, self-control, compassion, purity of intention, and gratitude—I was encouraged to practice these qualities not only on the yoga mat but also in the kitchen (and in life). Scrubbing black spots on pots became a meditation of scrubbing my mind of dark thoughts, controlling the urge to gossip silenced my mind to find inner peace; mopping the floor turned into an inspiration for humility; and blessing the food became a joyful expression of gratitude.

I always tell my students, "Your love is the most important ingredient in everything you make." Sometimes the best intentions still lead to a kitchen disaster, but your efforts will be appreciated because you sincerely tried your best. Cooking is an expression of love, a way of giving of yourself. We express love either through an act that creates life or through an act that sustains life. Let your loving energy charge the food you prepare so that the people who eat it will feel nurtured and healed. And keep in mind that nurturing, delicious, memorable meals that burst with vitality come from high-quality, wholesome, invigorating, sustainable real ingredients. However, let us not overlook another hidden energy behind the ingredients: the energy that comes from *you*. Your heart and mind carry unique vibrations that flow through your hands as you prepare the food. As you peel, chop, mix, and cook, your energy is colored by what you're thinking and feeling, and your thoughts are affected by what's happening to you outside of the kitchen. It is all connected and very personal, and it is all a part of our human evolution.

I put my heart into writing this book. Thanks to my many incredible teachers, I tried to present true knowledge of food and cooking and my personal experience of the application of that knowledge. I sincerely hope that between the lines and the recipes of this book you will discover the type of conscious Ayurvedic cuisine you can live with. It may begin with your intention to take better care of yourself and eat healthier. It may begin with swapping some ingredients and including lots of fresh seasonal vegetables and whole grains. Or it may affirm the journey of health and self-discovery you've already begun. We are all beginners at something, but it is a personal awakening that starts us on a path. If you feel that this book came to you at the right time, please keep it in your kitchen and use it daily. If the concepts of Ayurvedic cooking do not appeal to you at this time, then please put this book away where you can see it; may it draw you when the time is right.

Thank you for reading. Thank you for cooking and caring.

May our paths cross the way our minds did.

With love,
Divya Alter

THE SIX TASTES OF FOOD

TASTE	PHYSICAL EFFECTS	EMOTIONAL EFFECTS	PREDOMINANT IN FOODS
Sweet	**In balance:** nourishment, body building, energy **In excess:** congestion, sluggishness, edema, indigestion, obesity, diabetes, puffy eyes, oily skin, blackheads	**In balance:** love, pleasure, satisfaction **In excess:** greed, attachment, neediness, complacency, lethargy, laziness	Sweeteners, fruit juices, honey, rice, wheat and other complex heavy carbs, milk, cream, ghee, fish, meat, fats/oils, most root vegetables, most nuts, cucumber, most fruits, licorice, saffron, cardamom, cinnamon, tarragon
Sour	**In balance:** digestion, elimination, cleansing **In excess:** acidity, heartburn, ulcers, rashes, burning in the throat, chest, heart; indigestion, premature aging, muscle weakness	**In balance:** mental acuity, mental invigoration **In excess:** envy, resentment, regret, excessive criticism	Yogurt, cheese, green grapes, unsoaked raisins, citrus fruits, tamarind, tomatoes, vinegar, all fermented foods, miso, wine, strawberries, rose hips
Salty	**In balance:** circulation, appetite, digestion, stimulating; boosts all other tastes **In excess:** hyperacidity, high blood pressure, skin rashes, accelerated aging, inflammation, eye problems, swelling, obesity	**In balance:** mental ease, zest for life **In excess:** mental rigidity, greed, addiction	Sea salt, rock salt, sea vegetables
Bitter	**In balance:** detoxification, liver cleanser, blood purification, skin toner, weight loss, anti-inflammatory; antithesis of sweet **In excess:** depletion of bodily tissues, anemia, low blood pressure, constipation, cold, insomnia, vertigo, premature wrinkles	**In balance:** mental clarity, desire for change, insight, dispels illusion **In excess:** dissatisfaction, disillusionment, grief	Bitter melon, dark leafy greens (e.g. kale, chard, collards) bitter greens (e.g. broccoli rabe, dandelion greens), turmeric, goldenseal, dill, fenugreek, gentian root, neem, coffee, cacao/cocoa, nicotine
Pungent	**In balance:** appetizer, good metabolism, circulation, clears phlegm, antifungal, antibacterial, gives glow to skin **In excess:** acidic digestion, burning sensation, colitis, ulcers, diarrhea, redness of skin, skin rashes, broken capillaries, intense perspiration, insomnia, dehydration, excessive thirst	**In balance:** ambition, motivation **In excess:** irritability, hate, anger, aggression, jealousy, overstimulation	Onion, garlic, leeks, radishes, horseradish, turnips, mustard greens, ginger, chiles, cloves, asafoetida, cayenne, mustard seeds, black pepper, cumin, mace, paprika, marjoram
Astringent	**In balance:** increased absorption, heals wounds, stops bleeding, shrinks pores, less sweating **In excess:** slow digestion, gas, constipation, cramps, heart problems, dryness, excessive thirst	**In balance:** optimism, well-being, introspection **In excess:** fear, insecurity, self-absorption	Apples, pomegranates, pears, cranberries, unripe bananas, persimmons, artichokes, sunchokes, plantains, broccoli, Brussels sprouts, cabbage, cauliflower, celery, potatoes, kohlrabi, sprouts, spinach, eggplant, parsley, lettuce, mushrooms, beans, lentils, tempeh, quinoa, buckwheat, rye, green and black tea, nutmeg, rosemary, oregano, psyllium

SOURCES

SV AYURVEDIC DINING

Divya's Kitchen
www.divyaskitchen.com

INGREDIENTS AND PRODUCTS

Chandika
www.chandika.com
High-quality Ayurvedic remedies, personal care products, and ingredients: Soma Salt, sunthi, turmeric, and many more spices and masalas, cultured ghee, kulthi, rose buds, manjistha powder, and more

Dharma Smart / Lissa Coffey
www.dharmasmart.com
Ayurvedic cooking ingredients, skin care products, and more

Floracopeia
www.floracopeia.com
Pure rose water, essential oils

High Vibe
www.highvibe.com
Organic high-quality olive oil, ghee, coconut oil, spices, seaweed, olives, sweeteners, and more

Jovial Foods
www.jovialfoods.com
Organic einkorn (berries, flour, pasta); gluten-free flours

Mountain Rose Herbs
www.mountainroseherbs.com
Fair-trade, organic spices and herbs, including rose buds/petals, lavender, and jasmine

Natren
www.natren.com
Yogurt starter

Pratima Skin Care and Spa
www.pratimaskincare.com
Ayurvedic skin care products and spa treatments

Pure Indian Foods
www.pureindianfoods.com
Organic yellow split mung dal, chana dal, flours, cultured ghee, and more

The Yoga Farm
www.theyogafarm.com
Certified Organic compassionate farm for ahimsa dairy, whole grains, vegetables, honey, and more.

Poshan Foods
http://poshanfoods.com/
Organic ahimsa ghee and other products.

EQUIPMENT

Ancient Cookware
www.ancientcookware.com
Traditional Ayurvedic clay pots and other non-toxic natural cookware

SV AYURVEDA: KNOWLEDGE AND TRAINING

Bhagavat Life
www.bvtlife.com
SV Ayurvedic cooking classes and professional culinary training

Divya Alter's Recipe Blog
www.divyaalter.com

Vaidya R. K. Mishra
www.vaidyamishra.com

SV AYURVEDIC CONSULTATIONS

Dr. Marianne Teitelbaum
www.drmteitelbaum.com

ACKNOWLEDGMENTS

Twenty-six years ago, when my cooking journey began, I was young and green and did not speak a word of English. Today I am thrilled to celebrate not only the heights of my cooking career but also the completion of a book I wrote on a topic and in a language that were foreign to my upbringing. If that was possible for me, then imagine all the possibilities in your life!

Back in 2012, I started working on this book, and Kurt Opprecht and Andrea Wien helped me edit my first sample writing—thank you for bringing sense to it then! Sarah Jane Freymann, I could not have dreamed of a more experienced and enlightened literary agent. Thank you for believing in me as an author and for opening the door to the publishing world for me. Ellen Scordato, you cradled me as my writing mentor, consultant copyeditor, and friend from the first to the last word in this book and beyond—I'm most grateful to you. Martynka Wawrzyniak, you are an angel and a warrior among acquisition editors. Thank you for including me in the Rizzoli family, for your expert guidance in the production of the book, and for your kind friendship—you've changed my life more than you can imagine. Christopher Steighner, Rizzoli Senior Editor and head of the cookbook division, your editorial advice was invaluable. Rizzoli Publisher Charles Miers—I'm so grateful for your expertise in making this book the best it can be. Thank you, dear Leda Scheintaub, for your guidance and superb copyediting. William and Susan Brinson with the assistance of Stephanie Munguia: your exquisite photography deserves an award. To my food stylist, Micah Morton, and prop stylist, Sarah Smart—thank you for making the food look so attractive and achievable. Jan Derevjanik, I'm so grateful for your elegant graphics and design.

Heartfelt gratitude to my friends who supported this book financially: The Max and Sunny Howard Memorial Foundation, Naomi Sinnreigh, Pratima Raichur, Rosemarie Sepulveda, Britton Nohe-Braun, Rikin Patel, Paul and Lenka Knag, Hayes Holderness, Joshua Greene, Gunagrahi Goswami, Linda Gim, Teri Covington, Sarvenaz Bakhitiar, Emi and Phil Murray, Julie Hall, Dr. Julian Raymond, Jessica Leffler. You generosity inspires me to pay it forward.

What to Eat for How You Feel also grew with the nurturing support of my dear friends Shalom Harlow, Michael Halsband, Chef Heather Carlucci, Aracely Brown, Jimmie Stone, Jose N. Garcia, Katia Laine, Tiagi Lambert, Kandarpa Buckory—thank you for illuminating me with your brilliant minds and compassionate hearts.

The following friends assisted as test readers and recipe testers: Vaidya R. K. Mishra, Dr. Pratima Raichur, Vishakha Devi, Joshua Greene, Amanda Wahlstrom, Federica Norreri, Ryan Schmidt, Sara Wafia, Eileen Millan, Bijal Shukla, Madhurya Shroff, PJ Mark, Dr. Leonore Tiefer, Gina Dimant, Lisa Angerame, Wojciech Krakowski, Michelle Reyf. Your insights helped me improve the text and ensure that the recipes work—thank you profusely!

I could not have cooked the many dishes for the food photography without the kind help from Lauren Tremaine, Karen Marmorato, Suzanne Von Eck, Jose Cruz, Florence Swanstrom, Ellen McCormick, Lauren Suarez, Tanya Kuhn, Tamalyn Miller, Patricia Boyle, Parvita Jain, and Jennifer Madrid—my gratitude to you all.

Special thanks to the following companies for so graciously lending us props for the photography at no cost: Fefo Studio, Blackcreek Mercantile, and Sarah Kersten Studio.

To my Ayurvedic teachers, Vaidya R. K. Mishra, Dr. Marianne Teitelbaum, and Jaidev Singh: your presence and teachings transformed my life, improved my health, and enlightened my being. I can only express my profound gratitude to you through service.

To my spiritual mentors, Krishna Kshetra Swami (Dr. Kenneth Valpey), Bhakti Tirtha Swami, and Dravida Dasa, and to my cooking mentor Yamuna Devi: thank you for your unconditional loving guidance, encouragement, and wisdom. I cannot imagine what my life would be had I not met you.

To my cooking class students who persistently asked me to put my recipes into a book—thank you for your eagerness to learn.

My close family cheered me on through every stage of the creation of this book. In Bulgaria, Mom (Vera Marinova), Dad (Naiden Naidenov), and sister Radka Naidenova—I hope one day you will hold this book in Bulgarian! Thank you, Papa (Nick Alter) and Mom (Julia Alter) for loving me the way I am. And to the person I appreciate and get to cook for every single day, my husband, Prentiss Alter: your wisdom, loving tolerance, relentless optimism, sharp intelligence, and perceptive palate help me be the best chef and human being I can be. Thank you!

What to Eat for How You Feel is my humble offering of love and gratitude to you all.

INDEX

First published in the
United States of America in 2017
by Rizzoli International Publications, Inc.
300 Park Avenue South
New York, NY 10010
www.rizzoliusa.com

© 2017 Divya Alter
Text © 2017 Karen Page

Design by: Jan Derevjanik

Rizzoli Editor: Martynka Wawrzyniak

Photography: William and Susan Brinson

All rights reserved. No part of this publication may be reproduced, stored in a retrieval system, or transmitted in any form or by any means, electronic, mechanical, photocopying, recording, or otherwise, without prior consent of the publishers.

2022 2023 2024 2025 / 15 14 13 12 11 10 9

Distributed in the U.S. trade by
Random House, New York

Printed in China

ISBN: 978-0-8478-5968-9

Library of Congress Control Number: 2016955624